S0-BDP-043

What You're Looking for is *Not* in the Fridge!

Samantha,
I hope you
enjoy!

Julia

What You're Looking for is *Not* in the Fridge!

How I Found Myself
When I Stopped Looking There

By Julia Grocki, MS, MA, RDN, LDN

New Beginning Nutrition Counseling, LLC
Berwick, Pennsylvania

www.FightEmotionalEating.com
www.notinthefridge.com

What You're Looking for is Not in the Fridge!
How I Found Myself When I Stopped Looking There
Copyright 2017 by Julia Grocki
All Rights Reserved. Printed in the U.S.A.

No part of this book may be used or reproduced in any manner
without written permission except in the case of brief quotations
embodied in critical articles or reviews. For information, contact the
author/publisher.

Library of Congress Control Number: 2017911738
Grocki, Julia.
What you're looking for is not in the fridge!: how I found myself
when I stopped looking there/Julia Grocki.

Paperback:
ISBN-13: 978-0-9992450-0-2
ISBN-10: 0-9992450-0-7

eBook:
ISBN-13: 978-0-9992450-1-9
ISBN-10: 0-9992450-1-5

Cover Art by Ann Kohut Williams.

To inquire about special discounts for bulk purchases of this book or
having the author speak at your live event, please contact Julia
directly at FightEmotionalEating@gmail.com.

Legal Statement

This work is not intended to diagnose any disease or other health issue. It is not intended to substitute for advice from your healthcare team. The author is not responsible for injury or loss resulting from the use of presented information.

The presented information is based on the author's life experience as well as research available to her at the time of publication. Mention of specific products or stores does not constitute endorsement. Each of the trademarks identified herein are the property of their respective owners, who have no endorsement, affiliation, or sponsorship with the author, this book, or its contents.

Nutrition Prescriptions

While mindful eating practice encourages you to listen to your body and eat what you would like, there are some health issues that prevent this from being an option. For example, if your physician or dietitian advised you to restrict or limit specific foods, such as if you have kidney disease or heart failure, please continue to do so. If you have been put on a fluid restriction by your physician continue to follow that advice as well.

Please note that mindful eating practice has been shown to result in better blood sugar control. Many people with diabetes think there are many foods they "can't" have. This is not true. If you learn to eat slowly, savor your food, and listen to how your body reacts to it, you will end up eating less, which may help you control your blood sugar.

Dedication

This book is dedicated to everyone who struggles with their relationship with food, especially to those who have shared their stories with me. You validated what I always expected, that I was not alone and that there are many more individuals that need help. Your vulnerability inspired me during difficult times, giving me the motivation to complete this work.

Contents

Acknowledgements

I have been talking about this book and working on it for years. I have received support and encouragement from too many people to name. If you think I mean you, you are right. "Thank you" will never seem like enough. You have helped me, and the many people I hope this book touches.

I am grateful that I have a big family who loves and adores me. I am lucky to have learned different things from every one of you. It is amazing how people who are related can be so different!

Throughout my life I have been blessed with an eclectic group of friends. Along with my family, you helped shape me into the person that I am today. I love you for that!

I have been a work in progress my whole life. I have always been trying to figure things out.... both how to be better for myself, and how to teach those around me so that they can feel better too. I admit I have often been too pushy. Thank you all for putting up with that.

Thank you to my clients. Working with you has validated that I have been on the right track. Thank you for being brave and sharing your stories with me. I appreciate the support you have given me for this endeavor as well.

Thank you to Amanda Otruba, Janet Smith, Carolyn Beach, and Sam Osborne for proofreading this work. I appreciate your time and feedback! And to Ann Kohut Williams, thank you for capturing the spirit of my book in your cover art!

Preface

This book took me years to piece together. It took twelve years from start to finish… to identify my food issues, record my feelings as I healed, return to school to become a dietitian and finish polishing it up. It is obvious that I mostly recorded the painful parts of my life. I wanted to let my readers know, especially my friends and family, that my life has not all been pain. I have been as high as I have been low. I have many fond memories of growing up… dancing in the kitchen with my Mom to Motown classics as she ironed clothes, watching action movies with my Dad, playing the player piano in the basement at my grandparents' house, hanging out with my Pop and learning how to use his tools, spending a lot of time at both grandparents' houses, hanging out with our cousins, walking downtown with my uncles, hiking with my aunt and siblings to collect water samples and inspect them under her microscope, reading library books under the beautiful maple tree in her yard, craft projects, Friday nights trolling around the mall or going to sports events with my girls, weekly taco night at my buddy's house, listening to friends play music on the porch, cross-country practices and races, parties, hanging out with my Gram on her front porch, chatting it up with my aunt and uncles, and lots of sleepovers and giggling. I have many fond memories as an adult as well. My good memories could fill a book too, but that isn't the focus of this one. This book describes how I got through the darkness until I came back to those bright times. Even in my darkest moments, there were bright spots… the time spent with friends and family that kept me fighting to figure this stuff out. I love you all and I thank you for those bright times.

Julia Grocki (July 2017)

Over the years a lot of people have tried to tell you what to do, especially when it comes to food. You've had a lot of voices in your head to sort out... to try to decide who is giving you the best information. What I mostly hope to accomplish with this book is to teach you how to start to listen to the voice you can learn the most from... your own.

Introduction

Ever find yourself wandering around your kitchen aimlessly? You open your cabinets and search the shelves. Then you go to your fridge, open it and stare. It has happened to most of us. You might have done it right before you sat down with this book. Personally, I've done more squats in front of the fridge than I have in the gym. I was looking for "something" and I knew it had to be in there somewhere. We know we are hungry, but often what we are hungry for is not food.

I wasn't in tune with what I needed or wanted for most of my life. Even if I did know, I didn't let myself want whatever it was for fear of not getting it. All I knew for certain was that I didn't like me. I kept turning to food for comfort or company, and it always let me down in the end. I'd eat, feel good about it briefly, but then hate myself a little bit more every single time. Over and over I did this, for years and years. I buried myself under shame, guilt and pounds of fat.

I didn't realize I had a problem with food. I considered my thoughts normal for someone who "should be" losing weight. In fact, this book didn't start as a book about my relationship with food. It started as a recording of my journey as I learned about how Polycystic Ovary Syndrome (PCOS) affected my life, and how I dealt with it. Surprisingly, my writing for an entire year revolved around my disgust with my inability to control myself around food. It had little to do with PCOS!

This book became about my life as I fought emotional and mindless eating. I lost a massive amount of weight over the years, but more importantly I learned how to be kinder to myself and soothe myself without food. It shows how I've maintained my weight despite being tested with many difficult life circumstances. In the past, I would have tried eating myself through most of my stress, pain, and sadness, gaining weight in proportion to how terrible I felt. As I went through the process of healing, I became empowered and realized I could help others overcome similar issues. It inspired me to return to school to become a dietitian and focus my studies on how to help others build a healthy relationship with food.

The more I wrote, the more I realized that this book is about becoming a stronger, confident, decisive, more productive, healthier version of myself. Hopefully, this work will inspire you to do the same. It will help you start distinguishing between your body's signals that it needs fuel as opposed to other reasons you eat. You'll learn about yourself and what you need, and eventually discover that you need food less often than you think.

What I've written about is not just theory or research I've done; I've applied it all and I'm living proof that it works. I've been on this mission for a long time. I've wanted to let people know they have the power to change their lives. ***When the end goal seems impossible, most of the time our biggest obstacle is our disbelief.***

I recently watched one of those TV shows where the contestants have a lot of weight to lose, usually a hundred or more pounds. The winner is the one who can lose the most weight. They show people with personal trainers putting in long hours at the gym, doing extreme amounts of cardio and weight training. Often these people have time off from work and are in a "camp"-like setting where all they focus on is weight loss. They have people show them what to eat and often have meals prepared for them. They change many behaviors in their lives drastically. And yes, by the show's end, which for us could be an hour or two, but for them could be a year or so, they have lost an incredible amount of weight.

Hi all! My name is Samantha Smith!

I am a soon to be junior studying Nutritional Sciences here at Penn State.

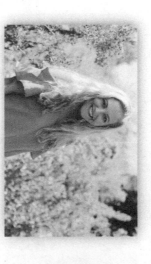

Follow me on
Instagram!
@sideofsamantha

Personal account:
@samanthacs

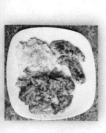
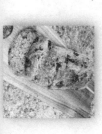
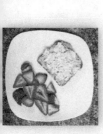
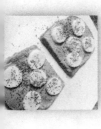

It is so hard to eat healthy in college while trying to maintain good grades, keep up with extracurriculars, and have no money. I know, I feel you!! So my blog gives some helpful tips and advice for eating healthy on a college budget. Head over to Sideofsamantha.com to check it out!

Hi all! My name is Samantha Smith!

I am a soon to be junior studying Nutritional Sciences here at Penn State.

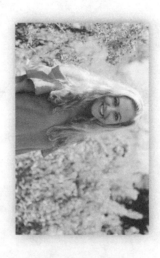

Follow me on Instagram!
@sideofsamantha

Personal account:
@samanthacs

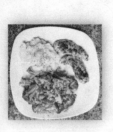
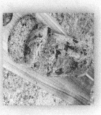
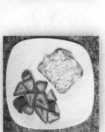
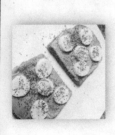

It is so hard to eat healthy in college while trying to maintain good grades, keep up with extracurriculars, and have no money. I know, I feel you!! So my blog gives some helpful tips and advice for eating healthy on a college budget. Head over to Sideofsamantha.com to check it out!

Hi all! My name is Samantha Smith!

I am a soon to be junior studying Nutritional Sciences here at Penn State.

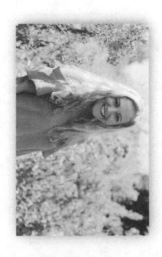

Follow me on Instagram! @sideofsamantha

Personal account: @samanthacs

It is so hard to eat healthy in college while trying to maintain good grades, keep up with extracurriculars, and have no money. I know, I feel you!! So my blog gives some helpful tips and advice for eating healthy on a college budget. Head over to Sideofsamantha.com to check it out!

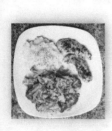

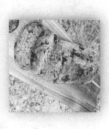

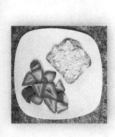

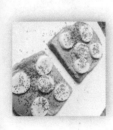

Hi all! My name is Samantha Smith!

I am a soon to be junior studying Nutritional Sciences here at Penn State.

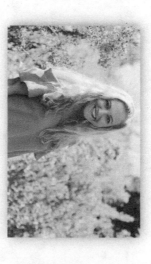

Follow me on Instagram!
@sideofsamantha

Personal account:
@samanthacs

It is so hard to eat healthy in college while trying to maintain good grades, keep up with extracurriculars, and have no money. I know, I feel you!! So my blog gives some helpful tips and advice for eating healthy on a college budget. Head over to Sideofsamantha.com to check it out!

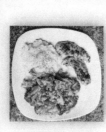

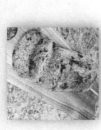

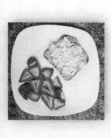

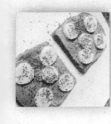

Hi all! My name is Samantha Smith!

I am a soon to be junior studying Nutritional Sciences here at Penn State.

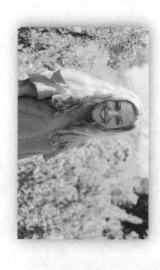

Follow me on Instagram!
@sideofsamantha

Personal account: @samanthacs

It is so hard to eat healthy in college while trying to maintain good grades, keep up with extracurriculars, and have no money. I know, I feel you!! So my blog gives some helpful tips and advice for eating healthy on a college budget. Head over to Sideofsamantha.com to check it out!

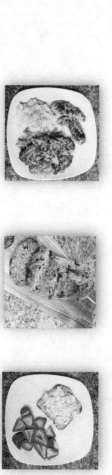

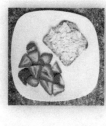

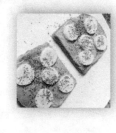

Hi all! My name is Samantha Smith!

I am a soon to be junior studying Nutritional Sciences here at Penn State.

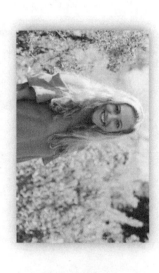

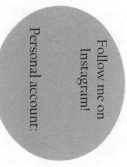

Follow me on
Instagram!

Personal account:

It is so hard to eat healthy in college while trying to maintain good grades, keep up with extracurriculars, and have no money. I know, I feel you!! So my blog gives some helpful tips and advice for eating healthy on a college budget. Head over to Sideofsamantha.com to check it out!

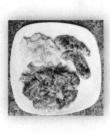

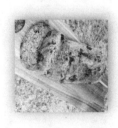

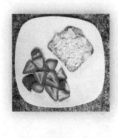

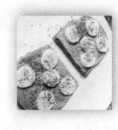

Hi all! My name is Samantha Smith!

I am a soon to be junior studying Nutritional Sciences here at Penn State.

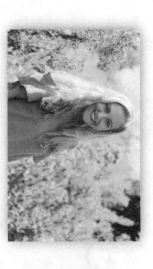

Follow me on Instagram!

Personal account:

It is so hard to eat healthy in college while trying to maintain good grades, keep up with extracurriculars, and have no money. I know, I feel you!! So my blog gives some helpful tips and advice for eating healthy on a college budget. Head over to Sideofsamantha.com to check it out!

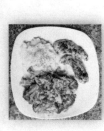

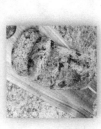

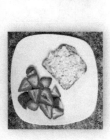

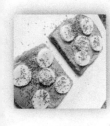

I don't want you to think that you require the same circumstances to achieve better health, including weight loss. You don't need to exercise eight hours a day, have chefs prepare healthy meals, and take time off from work, while being removed from your daily stressors. All you need to do is change one thing at a time, practice it and make that new behavior stick. Then you can decide what you want to do next. I've made small changes over time and have succeeded in keeping off 130 pounds over the last twelve years.

I started my journey as a frustrated 25-year-old woman who weighed 350 pounds. I was depressed, with low self-esteem and no energy at all. Today I'm fit and confident. I have armed myself with an array of coping mechanisms to help me deal with life's stressors instead of turning to food. I did this while working full time and wearing many other hats, like we all do. I lost weight in real life, not in a bubble. I continue to find new things I'd like to change. I work on those behaviors and I become stronger and healthier all the time. You can do this too!

I know you've heard that eating well is good for you. You understand your current lifestyle is probably making you sick. I also know you feel powerless. You feel like you cannot stop feeding your face. The more people tell you to stop, the more you want to do it. I know what it feels like to have your hand in the bag of chips and intellectually know you need to stop eating, that your health and future depends on it, but you know you won't stop until the bag is empty. You don't have to feel that helplessness, anger and worthlessness. You can take steps to start to build a healthy relationship with food today.

You may feel that the advice in these pages sounds too good to be true. 'Yeah, sure… I'll stop dieting. That will fix it!' Over time, it will! Trust me, I thought it was absurd too until I tried it. Nothing else has worked long-term for you, right? How many different diets have you tried that have failed you? How many pounds have you lost and regained over the years? Why not address your relationship with food and see where it takes you, instead of trying yet another diet that's bound to fail?

I started to realize I had a problem with food when I was 22 years old, but it took me quite a while to find the resources to help me move forward. I felt completely lost and had no idea what to do about it. Here is a sample of one of my earliest journal entries. When I wrote this entry I was a senior in college, studying chemistry. I completely freaked out the night after I skipped my first chemistry lab. See if you can relate...

Spring 2000

The minute I woke up today all I could think was that I didn't want to go to lab. I couldn't put that lab coat on... the one that doesn't fit. No, it's not that it doesn't fit from last semester, it's the one I bought to replace the one that doesn't fit from last semester, and it doesn't fit either. It's the biggest size they've got, and it doesn't fit! Every Tuesday that is the ONLY THING I think about. Today I let it win. I skipped lab. Never pulled that one before. What's the sense of going if I don't even think about what I'm doing while I'm there? Sometimes I worry I may hurt someone or myself.

I slept until noon. Then I ate almost a whole half gallon of ice cream. Then I ate half of a pizza. I will just eat whatever is in front of my face. It's like a habit. I don't feel like I can control it. Food is all I think about. Last night I tried to read Aristotle for Philosophy class. Every two or three lines or so I thought "I want some ice cream" or "I want some party mix". I

WASN'T EVEN HUNGRY! I don't know if I'm ever actually hungry. Why should I be?! I EAT ALL THE TIME!!!

It's like if I eat and nobody knows or remembers the food was in the house… if I hide it, then it's ok. One time I went to get coffee for my buddy and me and I scarfed down two donuts before I got back to the house, which is only two blocks away! I do it all the time. Then I try to convince others, and myself, that I didn't eat all day. I think that is what I tell people so that we all believe it, so I won't feel as bad for finishing my plate or getting dessert.

I've cried for the last two weeks. I feel so helpless. I cry as I write this. I don't know what to do. I don't know how this happened. I don't know why my reflection doesn't look like me anymore. HOW DID I LET MYSELF GAIN 80 POUNDS BACK?!! WHO IS THIS FAT GIRL AND WHAT DID SHE DO WITH JULIE?!!

If I can't keep promises to myself, how can I keep them for anyone else? Why should anyone trust me? I lied to the chair of my department today. I've lied to all of my professors as to why I've missed classes. I didn't think "I'm sitting home eating, crying and sleeping" would fly. I've lied to my family. I've lied to my friends. I've lied to myself. I don't feel like I can stop eating on my own. I feel like I sound crazy. I don't want my friends and family to find out.

I thought that the days of painting a smile on my face were over. I thought that once I had lost weight in high school I would continue to be happy and never have to pretend again. My act is so good that a few classmates asked me what the heck I'm so happy about all the time. I wonder if they'd believe how often I cry. Pretty impressive act I can put on, huh?

I cry all the time. I cried in front of my mentor when my lab coat didn't fit. I cried when we got on the plane last week and my butt barely fit in the seat and my thighs were spilling over into my friend's seat. I cried when I could barely fit into the booth at the school cafeteria. I cried when I got caught in the desk at school. I cried when I had no clothes to wear for Christmas. I cried when the jacket I bought from UVA didn't fit; it was the largest size.

As I sit and write and cry I am still thinking about food. There is some pizza and ice cream left. My brain keeps responding "SURE!! Why don't you go eat the whole thing you fat loser! What the heck is wrong with you!?!'

I've been killing myself slowly with food. I know this. I can't stop. I don't know what to do. I can read Aristotle. I can figure out organic chemistry reaction mechanisms. But, I can't figure out how to stop eating. I feel like this food problem is controlling my whole life. I can't go on like this. Maybe someone else can figure this out for me. But who? I've got to try to get some help.

When I got done writing this I got up and went to the fridge. I know I'm not hungry. I can't be hungry. Why do I keep doing this?!

What I was looking for is not in the fridge…. never was.

Shortly after writing that entry I began to read about eating disorders. I sounded like half of a bulimic. I did not purge and didn't intend on starting. One time I knelt by the toilet after eating a whole quart of chicken and broccoli. I stayed down for a while contemplating it. I couldn't go through with it. I hated vomiting. For a while I called myself a "non-puking bulimic". I didn't know what to do with that. I didn't think it was a real diagnosis, so I ignored it and continued overeating and beating myself up. Why bother trying to figure out something that doesn't even have a name? I decided I was weak and there was probably nothing I could do about that. I pushed it aside until I crossed paths with someone who told me about emotional eating three years later. Regardless of whether you've been diagnosed with an eating disorder or disordered eating patterns, if you see yourself or loved ones in that journal entry please keep reading.

Throughout this book the terms food addiction, emotional eating, bingeing, compulsive eating and overeating will be used interchangeably. Regardless of what you call it, the healing process is the same. I didn't develop the methods I used to heal my relationship with food. When introduced to the phrase "emotional eating", I started reading everything I could find about disordered eating patterns. Many of the books give similar advice. With a lot of practice and determination, it actually worked! I came to learn that what I was practicing was considered "mindful eating". That phrase did not appear until years after I started my own journey, but it is what I teach my clients now.

I summarize the important steps I took to start building a healthy relationship with myself and with food. If you want additional information, I highly recommend reading books by authors listed in the back of this one. The concepts presented here are simple, but the practice is challenging until you fight long enough to rewire your thought processes. I describe the struggle as I fought through it, but

I am proof that it gets easier over time. That is why I share my journal with you.

First, I will take you through the early part of my life when I started to use food to cope. As I mentioned earlier, I have an endocrine disorder called PCOS, which affects one out of ten women in the U.S. Odds are you know someone who deals with the symptoms, so I give you a brief overview of this disorder. Then I explain the concepts of food addiction, emotional and mindless eating. That's how the book goes, back and forth between letting you inside my brain and showing you the steps I took to get to where I am today. If you are feeling adventurous, turn the page to start reading my story. Hold on… it's been quite the ride!

Chapter 1
The Tilt-A-Whirl Begins

My life has been like a Tilt-A-Whirl. You know what a Tilt-A-Whirl is, right? It's that carnival ride that spins around in a circle. The individual part you sit in spins, and the whole time you spin the whole thing tilts back and forth. Nothing made sense. How did I get here? I could look up and see my surroundings briefly, but my life spun so fast that I couldn't see how I fit in. At 20 years old I was happy, healthy, focused, goal-driven and ready to take on life. In what seemed like the blink of an eye five years passed; I was depressed, sickly, 350 pounds, exhausted, confused and not sure if I could get out of bed. I didn't know how to move forward. My path was blurry. Every time I looked up to focus I saw something different. I felt like that for quite a while.

I finally realized that if my life were like a Tilt-A-Whirl I could control the spinning. You influence the individual car of a Tilt-A-Whirl by how you lean into it. If you lean with the spin, you can spin faster; if you lean away from the spin, you can spin slower. *Every day I had choices to make that could slow down some of the spinning.* However, I knew it would take a long time to get off my Tilt-A-Whirl completely since this spinning and tilting started at a young age.

"Too Fat" Started Early in Life

As early as kindergarten I knew I didn't fit in. I was bigger than all the other kids. I couldn't move as well as my classmates in gym. I don't remember feeling bad about it until we had a square dance. I didn't find any cute clothes in my size that looked as nice as the other girls. Five years old and already afraid none of the boys would dance with me. It is sad, but that is one of my only memories from that year.

I was nervous going to a new school in first grade. I wanted to fit in. My Mom curled my long hair one day. I felt so pretty. When I got to school one of the boys called me Miss Piggy. He said all I needed were the ears. I popped him one. That was one of the only times I got called to the principal's office. I had to promise not to do it again. Well, next time I wasn't gonna let myself get caught. Who would stick up for me if I didn't?!

I started to wear a bra when I was in third grade. My friends thought that it was cool because I was "becoming a woman." I thought it sucked because it meant that I was too fat. I remember going to the pediatrician with Mom and hearing him tell her I was too heavy for my age. He gave her a list of foods I could eat to reduce my calories - cottage cheese, grapefruit, celery sticks and carrots. How did he expect a young girl to stick to a diet like that while watching all her friends eat cookies, pudding snacks, cheese crackers and brownies? I'm grateful she didn't try to put me on that diet, but I do remember the many conversations my pediatrician had with her about my weight. At 8 years old I knew I didn't like how I felt when I went to the doctors. Even worse, I was already uncomfortable in my skin.

The Start of my Emotional Eating

Many people have asked me if I remember when I started to eat emotionally. I avoided that question for a while since I didn't feel I had the right to talk about it. Today (3.4.13) my best friend Nikol gave me permission to tell her story... our story. She said I didn't have to protect her anymore. This wave of relief rushed over me. Intellectually, the 34-year-old me knew that I didn't have to protect her anymore, but the scared little girl inside me still felt like she did. Nikol was the first person I felt I had to protect... to save. There have been others after her. I guess I am still trying to save people, which is why I'm writing this book for you. So, I will continue to type tonight through my tear-blurred eyes.

In third grade I started using food to cope with life. Of course, I didn't realize it at the time. That's when my new friend Nikol let me know that her mom's boyfriend had been hurting her. He had been touching her in ways she shouldn't have been touched. Her mom didn't believe her. If her own mom didn't believe her, then why would my parents or any other adults? She made me promise not to tell anyone anyway. I didn't want to tell because I didn't want anyone to look at her differently. She felt ashamed. I felt ashamed for her. I wanted to protect her. I wanted my parents to protect her too. I wanted her to feel "normal" in my house… our house. She didn't have a father in her life, so I wanted to give her mine. She needed love, so I wanted to give her mine. The way I knew how to show love was the way I was taught… by giving her food.

I didn't grow up in an especially demonstrative house. I knew I was loved, but nobody ever said it. We did give each other food though. Family gatherings were centered around food, like in most homes; looking back I see that we ate a lot. After school time at my grandparents' house revolved around the snack. My aunt would come home from school, talk about her day and have her snacks. I remember a lot of bread and butter being consumed by all. After work Pop would bring home cookies and fig bars and pass them out. It felt like his "I love you". When Mom came home from work to her parents' house we'd eat dinner. Her parents showed their love by having dinner for ready for Mom, my sister, my brother and me when Dad was on the road. At night when we left Gram and Pop's house we'd have a bedtime snack with Mom… cups of ice cream, cheese, pretzels, or salsa and chips. That was the time we spent alone with her, with food while watching TV. We never talked as much as we should have... or at least as much as I wanted to or should have myself. And, like many families, when we did chat, we didn't spend time talking about feelings or what to do about them.

Dad sold bakery supplies for most of my childhood. He usually traveled from Monday through Friday. When Dad joined us again on Friday, we got to go out to eat as a family. I remember going out for fast food when a popular restaurant had the "salad bar" with fixings for tacos and a pasta bar. I didn't eat much salad... I mostly remember the chocolate pudding. That outing meant family. It also meant a lot of overeating.

After Friday night's dinner, we'd do our grocery shopping. We'd get to pick out snacks for the weekend. Those treats were added to the goodies that Dad brought home. The bakers gave him delicious cookies, donuts, cakes, pies and breads. We would all hang out and eat together... including Nikol. She and I would often retreat up to my bedroom with a box of chocolate frosted cake donuts and a bottle of soda or milk. We were safe. My parents were home. She had her PapaMan (her nickname for Dad). We had our food. I knew she wasn't getting hurt. A few more friends often joined in. I started building an extended family at a very young age.

The thought of Nikol's mother's boyfriend's face makes me sick. I'm nauseous right now as I type. He violated my friend. He took things from Nikol she could never get back. He made her feel like she didn't matter. She didn't feel seen. She didn't feel like a priority. She didn't feel protected. I wanted to protect her and I felt as if I failed over and over. I'm sorry for that beautiful little girl, who would look at me with her big, brown, watery eyes. She looked so lost and helpless. My overall feeling of failure started at such a young age. Unfortunately, it would become a theme in my life for many years. I was wired to feel like a failure. Wired to feel like I had to protect people. Wired to carry guilt. I didn't know what to do with any of that, so I tried to "fix" it with food.

She and I discussed these issues many times. I told her that for years I carried around horrible guilt; I didn't stop her from being molested AND I gave her an eating disorder. I felt like I screwed up her life. I felt like I dropped the ball. I should have known better. I should have told someone. I shouldn't have let it continue. He hurt her for years. The 9, 10, 11, 12-year-old girl inside me sometimes asks, "Why didn't you stop him?" I don't think I have forgiven myself. I don't think I truly understand that it wasn't my fault. I can say the words, "it was his fault... he's the one who hurt her", but I hold onto the guilt. It is getting smaller, but it's still there. I've always been hard on myself. I am working on that in therapy. (Now, in 2015 as I re-read this chapter I can happily say I've worked through it and let it go. Counseling is a wonderful thing!)

Nikol and I would eat every chance we got. Her mom would leave chips (the green shiny bag of sour cream and onion... seeing that bag in the store still can stir something up inside me), hot dogs, Ramen noodles... lots of salty stuff in the apartment. She was rarely home. We'd hang out and eat everything. Ramen noodles are still one of my favorite comfort foods. In fact, I called a friend earlier and told him I had Ramen noodles for dinner and he asked me what was wrong.

Whenever we needed a sweet fix we'd head down to my house. We were always stocked up. We'd also go "work" at her Mom's place of business, doing odds and ends, like stuffing and licking envelopes for a few bucks. Then we'd take our earnings down to the corner store and stock up. Swedish fish, gummy worms, Tootsie Rolls, lollipops, fun dips, candy cigarettes, those awful-tasting colored dots attached to strips of paper in rows of four or five (What the heck was that about anyway? They were gross, tasted mostly like food coloring, yet I got them all the time!), bottle caps, those weird wax bottles with the sickening-sweet liquids in them.... the list goes on and on. We'd do anything they'd ask us to do to work for the junk food. So much candy and junk consumed over the years. *It never fixed the fact that she was getting hurt, but food was all we had, so we kept turning to it.*

Nikol was my best friend, my every day person. She went to her extended family's houses in the Midwest every summer. Part of me was happy that she could get away from the molester. The selfish part of me wanted her with me. Who would let me know if I had done a good job if she wasn't around? She was my helper and cheerleader. We didn't get to talk much since that was the time of long distance phone charges and calling cards. I didn't know how to deal with the sadness of her being gone, so I turned to food.

I feel like we lived in this secret world that the adults didn't know about… we flew under the radar as often as possible. She was getting hurt. I was feeling like a failure. We were trying to eat our way out of it.

Chapter 2
Hard on Myself for So Long

In grade school, I remember sitting at the lunch table and looking at everyone's food, wondering if they thought I ate too much. I tried to appear less interested in food. For example, if I had chips I would put some on each side of me on the table and ask one of the boys to arm-wrestle. The loser would have their hand smashed into the chips. What a waste of chips! For the record, I won quite a few times. I used to like it. Guess my competitive nature started young!

By fourth grade, I remember getting dressed up in leotards with my Mom and aunt to do Jane Fonda workouts. How many other girls out there have fond memories of childhood aerobics? Probably more than I think. I started fixating on my fat by fifth grade. I think I stood around five feet. I was the tallest in my class and in the 160-pound range. I shopped in the adult section and my mom shortened my pants, while my friends got to shop in the kid's section. I envied my friends who could shop anywhere. Thank God for Lane Bryant. That was the only store whose clothes I knew I could fit into, and more importantly, get clothes that didn't make me look like I was in my 70s.

Random Thought

Why is it that plus size departments are often filled with clothing with embroidered birdcages, butterflies, flowers and stuff? Is that so plus size women can blend in with the surrounding nature? I can imagine the talk in a plus-size designer's studio, "Let's stick an embroidered woodpecker on the leg since they look like tree trunks anyway!" Why don't skinny clothes have embroidered crap? Don't thin women want to blend in with nature too? Is it so plus size women can't possibly be mistaken for thin? Like if you were on the borderline of fat and skinny, people could tell you were fat if you turned around and had embroidered pictures of horses running through a meadow on your shirt?!

In case the embroidered crap isn't enough, the clothing manufacturers insist on putting the "W" at the end of a plus size tag. Is that so if you were feeling thin, fitting into your size 18s, and you went shopping, you would be reminded that you were overweight since you had to look for those 18Ws? The "W" in my mind stood for "What makes you think that you should be allowed to feel good since you are obviously overweight?!" Do larger men's clothing sizes have a big "M" at the end of the size to signify men's overweight status? Is there that cut-off size for men, like the jeans go from 38 to a 40M? If guys had the "M" on their size, they wouldn't have to wonder if they could be considered thin, the answer would be no!

And why does there have to be a "Women's" section? Women are women, no matter what their size. If the majority of us are overweight or obese, that means that more than half of us shop in the "Women's" section. Ironically, it means that all of us have the opportunity to feel less like a woman every time we go into a store. For example, you see pretty clothes that you'd love to try on, but then you get closer and realize your plus size butt is never going to fit into that size medium. Then you have to look up for the big sign that says "Women's", that says "Hey fat girl, you don't belong with the normal size girls! Get over here, isolated from the thin women where you belong". I remember feeling like that since middle school, and sometimes I still get ticked when I try looking in the women's section for clothes. But I digress; let me get back to middle school....

Exercise Started Young Too

During middle school, my family got a Nordic Track. The infomercial convinced me that it was the absolute most fun, easy, and beneficial workout. I pumped up my Bobby Brown, MC Hammer and TLC in the basement for a couple years doing the Track. I would work out for at least a half hour, 4 to 5 times per week. I felt more fit than ever. I thought I was so cool. My pants got bigger on me so I must have lost some weight, but that is about all I remember. And stop laughing at my music choices! It was the early 1990s after all. I still bust out those songs on occasion!

High School

I gained a lot of weight freshman year in high school. The transition to the new school was rough. I didn't like myself. I was uncomfortable with so many things… making new friends, interacting with boys, and trying to dress cute despite the lack of nice clothes in my size. I didn't want to walk down the hallway at times because I felt the judgment. Now I know that how I felt about myself wasn't too strange considering most teens aren't comfortable in their own skin. It was also the year my Gramma, my Mom's mother passed away. I'm sure we were all sad, although I don't remember anyone verbalizing it. I imagine I turned to food for comfort, but I don't remember specific incidents of bingeing that would have led to a lot of weight gain. I do remember that by sophomore year I reached 280 pounds. Of course, Gram passing happened before I was aware of my food issues. I didn't know that my behavior around food could have given me insight into how I felt. I had many years of mindless eating…. most of the time I wasn't paying attention to what, how or why I was eating.

It was hard for me to make it up the stairs at school, especially if I had to go from 1st floor to 3rd floor. It would take me a long time to recover; my heart would pound and I could barely catch my breath. I wouldn't want to talk for the first 10 minutes of class to prevent anyone from knowing how winded I had gotten. At the end of class I worried about whether the desk would get stuck to my gut. I'd try to wait until everyone left the classroom, pretending to pack up my bag, so I could get up without an audience. Unfortunately, that left me with less time to make it to the next class, causing me to hurry and be out of breath again.

Boys never looked at me unless they needed help with schoolwork, someone to pal around with or an easy target for their jokes. It made me feel very isolated since my girlfriends always seemed to have guys flirting with them. I wanted to be flirted with… to be noticed. I wanted to feel pretty, attractive, feminine. I thought I was cute when I looked in the mirror. Why didn't any of the boys seem to notice? Was my weight turning off every single boy I met?

I felt like nobody understood what I went through every day. I never tried to explain it to my friends, so now I know it was my fault I felt alone. As I look back, I see that I suffered from depression. I didn't know about it back then. I didn't think about telling anyone how I felt. I was sick a lot. In fact, I skipped school often that year, telling my parents I had diarrhea or vomiting. Most of the time it was true, but now I can see it was probably due to the extreme anxiety I felt from thinking about having to go to school.

I weighed 283 pounds the beginning of sophomore year. Not sure why I remember that number, but it is burned into my brain. I don't remember bingeing. Then again, I ate like my family ate, and many of them were overweight too. Alcoholism tends to run in families, so why not food addiction?

One of my friends and I had a tradition that we hung out at her house the night before the start of the new school year. The night before sophomore year her little brother called me a Sumo wrestler and I chased him around the block. I don't know what the heck I thought I would do if I caught him. It wasn't like we physically fought; we just used to pick on each other. He is five years younger than us and probably over 200 pounds lighter than me at that time. I would never have caught him. I don't know what possessed me. I remember being completely enraged. I'm sure it wasn't because of his one comment. It was probably due to the years of getting picked on, years of self-ridicule for not being able to change my appearance and years of trying to squash my feelings with food. As I chased him, I built up fierce momentum (which is directly related to mass, so go figure) running down the hill back toward the house. I fell and twisted my ankle so badly that my doctor said it would have been better to break it. I couldn't get around on crutches and missed the first several weeks of class. I was completely embarrassed that I didn't have the strength to carry myself around.

I had a lot of time to think at home. It seemed like a tragedy at the time, but it was one of the best things that ever happened. It is odd that a great gift could come in such an ugly package. At that point in my life I had reached a distinct fork in the road. I could either keep eating myself to death or I could take control of my weight and my life. I started to get excited thinking that I could take control. I started believing I could do anything if I wanted it enough, and I DEFINITELY wanted to lose weight! This is when my mental pep talks began.

My First Official Diet

I started a trendy low-fat diet. I thought I could eat whatever I wanted as long as the fat calories were 30% or less. The idea was that fat makes you fat. Yes, it is true that fat has 9 calories per gram and carbs and protein have 4 calories per gram. In theory, you could eat twice as many carbs and protein and come up with the same number of calories as by eating the same amount of fat. However, I didn't put a cap on my eating. I didn't pay attention to my physical hunger at all. I only ate "allowed" foods. The problem was that I ate ALL THE TIME. I found that many snack foods were under 30% calories from fat; I ate the heck out of licorice, any gummy candy, popcorn, breads, pastas, frozen yogurt, sorbet and low-fat snack cakes. That is something that I've observed many people do… seek out different versions of snack or "junk" foods that will fit within the current parameters of their latest fad diet. When I was on low-carb I found as many low-carb snacks as I could that I'd end up bingeing on. How much "cheesecake" made without sugar can a girl eat? You'd be surprised! Some diets have "free" foods. People often stock up on those free foods so that they have something to binge on when they are in the mood to overeat.

I ate everything low-fat, I exercised my butt off and I didn't lose much weight at all. That should have been a clue that this diet wasn't working very well. However, it felt good that I was eating "right". It felt good that I thought I was doing something right for the first time in my life.

I ended up developing a fear of all things greater than 30% in calories from fat. For years I didn't eat a single potato chip, candy bar, cake, pie or anything from a fast food restaurant if I didn't have the nutritional information and I could prove it was less than 30% fat. I ended up screwing myself up pretty badly. The paranoia that surrounded food became severe. People were proud of me for the "willpower" I displayed, but honestly, I was simply scared that those foods that didn't "fit" in my diet would make me gain all my weight back. That was my first official diet.

And the Running Begins

During spring of junior year in high school I started running. Ok, it was more like shuffling, but what do you want from an almost 260-pound girl? I started running because I wanted to be able to run the mile for gym class. The previous year I finished in what seemed like hours after everyone else, my face flush, sweat dripping, knees hurting and spots in front of my eyes. Everyone waited for me, staring. They all got up to walk back to the school. The finish line was a huge block away. I thought I would die before I made it back. Teenagers are dramatic. It's funny how now I don't recall who was in that gym class. I don't even remember my teacher. Bet they don't remember it either. At the time, I could have dug a hole and buried myself in it.

One day while shuffling down the street I heard a beep. It was a guy I did math with who happened to be a runner and other guys from the cross-country team. I figured it was another jerk who was getting ready to yell "fat ass" or something else derogatory. I've been "moo"ed at a lot... very creative! I got a call soon afterward from him about how he and the rest of the guys thought I should join the team. I thought they were nuts, but the more he talked, the more it sounded like fun. I felt like I was crazy, but I signed up the next day.

That summer we practiced every morning. What they considered "warming up" was faster and longer than I ever ran. It discouraged me. I wanted to shuffle right home. Somehow, I kept going back. It helped that there were a bunch of cute guys in little shorts, who were encouraging and supportive. Thanks guys! The coached amazed me too. They put as much effort into encouraging me, the girl who was bound to be last, as they did the fastest runners. They were always so proud of me and I pulled from their energy. I could never thank them enough for the impact that experience had on me.

By the end of the summer I ran the whole 3.1 miles. I got down to around 170 pounds. I'm 5'7" and I had a lot of muscle mass, so I looked pretty darn good. I got quite a big head. I got so strong that I could put my feet up on the arm of my couch and do pushups off it. I felt like my body floated as I walked. It is amazing what losing over one hundred pounds can do!

I absolutely loved cross-country. It was a wonderful experience. I also ran track that year, joined the cross-country team in college and ran all four years. My love affair with running is ongoing to this day.

First Sign of Polycystic Ovary Syndrome

One day while riding bikes in high school one of my best friends finally told me that he thought I should do something about my beard. What beard?! I didn't even realize I had one!!! I ran home and looked in the mirror and it looked like a bunch of peach fuzz. I thought everyone had a little peach fuzz! Then I got closer, turned to look from different angles, changed the lighting and saw that quite a few of these facial hairs were dark and long. I started plucking like crazy. The more I plucked the more hairs I saw. I didn't believe my eyes! Why the heck didn't anyone tell me sooner?! Sure, I thought he was a jerk for a little while; then I thanked him. I was glad to get rid of it so I didn't feel like I looked like a man. No wonder none of the guys saw me as dating material – I won their competition for beard-growing and didn't know it!

I talked with my family doctor about the facial hair. He thought it must run in my family. He never checked my hormone levels. Instead he referred me for electrolysis. Now there is a good idea! Let's take someone who is embarrassed about their excess hair, put them under a huge mirror and light, stick a sharp little needle in each follicle, zap it with a pulse of electricity, pluck the hair out and leave huge red bumps that last for days to draw more attention to her messed up face. Those freaking bumps didn't go away for days, even if I ran home, iced and then used the lotion they gave me. That lotion didn't match my skin tone, but was supposed to help cover everything up. Oh yeah, did I mention that each follicle needs to be zapped several times to work, and with all the growing time involved it takes over a year?! And who the heck has the cash for it when you're too busy buying food you shouldn't eat and magazines with diet tips? This leads me to another random thought...

Did you ever notice this one: magazines aimed at women are loaded with diet and exercise tips? "How to Lose 7 Pounds in a Week"; "Walk the Weight Off in Four Short Weeks" ... What the heck is a short week anyway? Seven days is seven days, right? "Lose Weight and Never Diet Again", etc. Right under the headlines are giant pictures of chocolate cakes drenched in raspberry sauce and whipped cream or cupcakes decorated like little farm animals you can make for your child's birthday party. So you look at the magazine, buy it for the weight loss advice, end up making the cupcakes for the child you don't have since you are infertile (another symptom of PCOS), and don't have enough time to decorate them since you're too busy, and then sit there and eat them all by yourself since you feel like shit about your weight, childlessness and the fact that you don't have enough time to do anything you want to do, like make frickin' piggies and duckies and crap out of the damn cupcakes... THEN... get a temporary sugar rush from the cupcakes, feel shittier then you did to start, wake up the next day and pick up a different magazine and start all over again. Sigh. Wait a minute... what the heck was I talking about? Ah yes, facial hair...

I've done it all... pluck, hot wax, wax strips, bleach, used depilatories. I finally started shaving my face and nothing else does it for me. Sure, the first time I did it I sobbed. Second time I did it I laughed. I wouldn't do it in front of anyone for years. I didn't mention it to people for a long time. Now I don't care who knows. If my facial hair bothers you, you've gotta find something more important to worry about. Mostly I like that at the start of the day I know my face is smooth. Anything besides shaving made me break out terribly. Then I would need tons of makeup to cover that up, which caused more breakouts. It's another vicious cycle. Some women with PCOS have trouble with acne, so irritating the inflamed skin isn't a good idea.

The more women I talk to about having to deal with facial hair, the more women admit that they have the same problem. We are mammals after all. We are covered in hair. Men happen to have more hair than women, but that doesn't mean that women should be expected to be entirely hairless! But, since that is the social convention, many of us find ourselves spending a lot of time on hair removal from many areas of the body. Why should removing hair on our face be more embarrassing than removing it from anywhere else?

I wish that my doctor tested my hormones when I went to him about the beard. Women generally do not have facial hair. A bell should have gone off that maybe something was physiologically wrong besides having crappy genes. I probably had high testosterone then from the PCOS and still have twice the upper limit for testosterone in women. [As I sit here and reread this several years later, I have testosterone right in the middle of the normal range for women, all from losing weight by doing what I describe in later chapters to repair my relationship with food. Woohoo!!!]

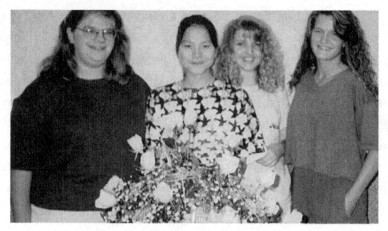

Celebrating with friends (1994)

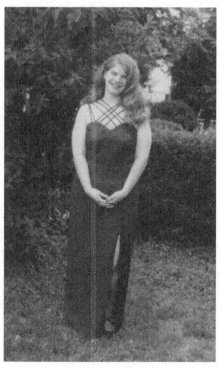

Senior Prom (1996)

My Weight Loss Success?

I wrapped up senior year on an incredible high. After losing 100 pounds I started coming out of my shell. I did things I had only wished I could do. I sang the National Anthem at all our high school basketball games. Me?! Solo... in front of everyone?! I performed in the school musical. I got a job and could stand on my feet after going to school all day. I started to like the person staring back at me in the mirror. It amazed me, but it "proved" that I could only "be me" if I were thin. It reinforced my belief that happiness was found on the number on the scale. I only maintained that loss for two years, along with the happiness and confidence.

Chapter 3
Dating, Gaining Weight, Falling Apart...
Then Off to Graduate School

Chet was my boss at the dollar store and I often talked to him, asking him for advice. I enjoyed going to work after school to unwind with my friend. Then suddenly I realized he was my guy... the one I went to all the time. The one that made me feel better. The one who listened. I enjoyed flirting with him. Was he flirting back? We had quite an age difference, but I felt comfortable around him. Several years after I worked with him, when he went on vacation for a week I realized how much I missed him. He had the courage to tell me he felt the same. First I thought it was nuts. I did a survey of my friends to see how they felt. I was mostly met with "you know how you feel, so why not give it a try." My Mom said the way I often talked about him it didn't surprise her. We started dating the summer before my senior year of college.

Chet was my first serious boyfriend. I was around guys all the time, but none of them showed any interest. Part of the attraction to Chet was that he gave me something I longed for for a very long time.... he made me feel like a girl. He made me feel pretty. He made me feel wanted and needed. He made me feel loved. Instead of cuddling up with my donuts at night, I got to cuddle up with him. For years I felt lonely. It always seemed as though my friends had someone. I'd often watch TV at night with a heavy heart and try to fix it with food. When I realized how good it felt to have someone in my life I dove right in without checking the depth of the water. We progressed quickly in our relationship.

Like most couples, our dates often consisted of going out to eat. We had a lot of fun together. It was natural to stop paying attention to what I ate and drank…. I simply enjoyed myself. I went out to eat all the time with my friends too. I ended up gaining thirty pounds by the end of the year. I stopped doing as many cross-country races since my knees ached and I started feeling fatigued. I felt like a lazy sack since I started slacking on everything. I comforted myself with food. I gained more weight… became less active… felt bad… ate more… and repeat. Notice a theme forming? Too bad I didn't. Later I would find that there was another underlying cause to my exhaustion.

December that year I got sick and almost passed out after staying up all night doing math homework. I went to the ER and my temperature was 104 degrees. They said they didn't know what was wrong, and I must have "an infection" since my white cell count was up. No foolin'! The fever could have been a clue, huh?! I was worn out for the rest of the semester. I remember staring at the letter "I" on a molecule and wondering why the heck someone would put that on a chemical structure. I completely forgot that "I" stood for iodine. That was crazy since I learned the symbol for iodine in middle school.

I was extremely tired over winter break. I ended up back in the ER with a fever and a rash over my torso. They couldn't figure out what was wrong with me. They wanted to do a spinal tap to check for meningitis, which I found ridiculous since I didn't have any other symptoms besides the fever. I didn't let them do the test. They even tested me for HIV. They couldn't find anything wrong besides the white count. Then I got strep throat three months in a row. The third time was in April. I ended up seeing a different doctor. He said that because my lymph nodes were swollen, I had the spots on my throat, and the constant fever that he thought I had mononucleosis. He did a mono spot and I did indeed have mono. He speculated that I had it since December and my tests didn't pick it up. Great news! I had mono for four months and didn't know it! YAY!

(Sarcasm runs in my family.) I kept trying to push myself through it since I thought I had just become fat and lazy. By that time I gained a total of 50 pounds. I could barely make it to my classes and didn't have enough energy to do my project for my thesis.

I had a lot of time to think while I lay around, unable to do my homework or anything else. I started to acknowledge an obsession with food and my weight. That is when I wrote the journal article I included in the introduction to this book. I talked to the chair of my department about the mono, my low energy levels and depression, and he granted an extension on my thesis defense. I talked to my doctor about the food issues and depression and he gave me Welbutrin to take. It was supposed to help my depression. It was originally to help smokers quit, so he hoped it would help me with the food cravings. I guess he didn't understand how emotional eating worked or he would have recommended a counselor who dealt specifically with that issue. I ended up going for counseling the summer before I went to Virginia. I only talked about the depression and not about the food. I didn't continue with it when I got to Virginia. Somehow, I managed to push my awareness of my food issues to the side. Obviously, it continued to serve a purpose.

Graduate School

I was accepted to University of Virginia (UVA) for graduate school in the middle of all this mess. I had been excited to go, especially since Chet asked me to marry him and agreed to move with me. But, by the time we moved my confidence had been shattered. My grades for the last year of undergrad were poor and I wrecked my GPA. My moods were all over the place with the Welbutrin. My enthusiasm fizzled to nothing. I started withdrawing from most of my friends. I started to feel like a failure... yet again.

I defended my thesis and passed in the middle of July 2000. Chet and I moved to Virginia the following week. We managed to pick out a house, buy it, close on it, clean it, pack everything, move and unpack it, all within two weeks. My friends and family helped, but that was a lot to do in that time period. I was probably still recovering from the mono since I had worn myself down over the previous six months. I exhausted myself.

The first few weeks at UVA were terrible. I couldn't concentrate. I slept a lot. I couldn't make it to all my classes. When I did make it to class, nothing made sense. I didn't have enough energy to do my homework or grade my students' lab reports. I would read one line and end up closing my eyes. I would read the next line and repeat. I would have to start over by the time I got to the end of the page because I couldn't remember what I read. I tried reading magazines or things on the Internet; I couldn't even do that. I didn't have enough energy to teach lab. I couldn't walk around the lab for long. It drained me. I ached so badly I ended up icing my knees and falling asleep as soon as I got home. I'd fall asleep with my feet propped up on the wall trying to drain the fluid that collected.

I got a 30% on my first organic chemistry exam. I couldn't believe it since it was my favorite chemistry. I knew graduate school would be difficult, but I also knew I wasn't myself. I knew I had to take time off, which maybe I should have done in the first place. They were supportive at UVA. They said I could finish teaching chemistry lab for the semester and I could come back the following fall semester.

And as if I didn't feel bad enough…

I had diarrhea the whole previous year, but it got worse when I decided to take the time off. Chet and I would go out to dinner, then go shopping or to a movie or something and I would end up getting horrible stomach cramps. I'd have to run to the nearest bathroom, possibly several times. Then I would want to go home. I remember eating on a boardwalk once and trying to walk down the beach. We practically had to run back. I felt like I wouldn't make it in time. Usually I would have to eat hours before we wanted to go somewhere so I could get done being sick to my stomach before we left the house.

I ended up seeing a doctor at the school. He diagnosed me with Irritable Bowel Syndrome (IBS) and told me to add more fiber. I thought fiber relieved constipation, but he explained that it would bulk things up so they wouldn't have to leave my body so quickly. It sounded logical to me. I followed his advice and it helped. All that time I suffered with chronic diarrhea and all I had to do was add more fiber. I couldn't believe it! Other doctors told me anxiety caused it and I had to relax. I'm sure that was part of it. I'm not convinced I had true IBS since I never had those symptoms again, but I'm sure glad this fiber thing worked out well!

Chronic Fatigue Syndrome?!

I told the same doctor about my aches and pains, low energy, memory loss and depression. He diagnosed me with Chronic Fatigue Syndrome (CFS), after doing a bunch of blood work to rule out other problems. They said CFS didn't have a cure and all I could do was cope. I read all these books about it and they said the same thing. There were discouraging stories about people having to quit their jobs. Nobody would believe them. People thought that it was all in their head. I didn't want to accept that it could happen to me. At that time I was exhausted and didn't try too hard to find another explanation. I rolled with the CFS diagnosis for a couple months. All that time I felt exhausted and lazy. I looked for energy and comfort and I turned to food again. I was stuck in that eat, feel bad, gain weight, eat more, feel even worse and repeat cycle.

What the heck is a Dermoid?!

In December 2000, I started having pelvic pain on my right side. I got set up with a gynecologist. He told me he felt something during my pelvic exam and ordered an ultrasound. They saw "something" on the right ovary and told me my doctor would contact me. I waited weeks until I finally heard what that "something" was since my doc was out of town for a while. I had dermoids on both ovaries. The one on the right was "pretty big" and he thought they better come out. There was a chance I could lose my ovary. I was scared. It was especially scary when I went to the Internet to find out about dermoids. They are growths made up of skin, fat and sometimes hair and teeth. They had a small chance of being malignant. A small chance is still a chance, and it terrified me. I had a couple dreams of this little monster inside that was going to eat me from the inside out. I wanted them out.

I read about PCOS while looking up info about ovaries and talking with one of my counselors. By this time, I saw several different counselors since every medical doctor told me that my symptoms were all in my head. My "alternative medicine" doctor recommended that I have my hormones tested in my saliva. The saliva testing gives the level of "free" hormones, those that are not bound to anything else in the body and are therefore free to perform their duty. Those results showed very high testosterone, and the "female" sex hormones showed I wasn't ovulating, releasing an egg during my period. These results plus the fact that I had facial hair, absent periods, weight gain, acne, etc. led me to believe I had PCOS.

I told my gynecologist that I thought that I had PCOS. He didn't think I had it. He thought I was "just depressed and eating too much". So, I simply should "stop eating so much". Well f@#% you very much doctor… I mean thank you very much for the enlightening advice. I also asked him if he thought the dermoids could have screwed up my ovaries, and in turn, my hormones got out of whack. He told me they were asymptomatic, meaning they would have no effect on me. He didn't think my body could have been thrown off by having my ovaries all stretched out and wrapped around tumors?! Oh, that makes a whole heck of a lot of sense. But, since I was out of my mind at that time I said, "Duh, ok, you must be right, take the dermoids out and I will stop eating so much."

It didn't work.

The dermoids were the size of a softball and a golf ball. The gynecologist said if they got bigger they would twist things around down there and that is why they should come out. My ovaries, a major part of the endocrine system (hormone system), were stretched out. You can't tell me that they did not affect my hormonal balance. The tumors themselves were shown to release different hormones by several research groups. They release hormones! I asked if they would have anything to do with my PCOS and several doctors said there was no relationship. Logic tells me that if these tumors released hormones AND messed up my ovaries' structure, that my whole hormonal symphony could have been thrown off balance. Therefore, as far as I'm concerned, they could have made my PCOS worse. I guess there is no way to prove it.

I ended up getting the dermoids removed in the summer of 2001 and it was a long, hard recovery. They could not do a laparoscopic procedure because of my weight. That's where they pump your abdominal cavity with gas to give them room to work and only have to make small slits in your body. They use a little camera to see inside. The recovery is quicker. Instead they gave me a six-inch "bikini" cut under my large stomach fat roll. All I could think when he told me the name of the cut was 'Well thank God I'll be able to wear a bikini someday!', while picturing stuffing my over 300-pound body into a few strips of fabric. The surgery site got infected and the entire surrounding area was yellow and hard as a rock after a few days. I never saw anything like it and feared my skin would never go back to normal. It did indeed go back to normal in time, but it was months before I felt ok.

I got a urinary tract infection after the procedure. That was not fun. I couldn't stand up out of my recliner by myself. Chet had to help me every time I went potty. I went every five minutes. I would squeeze out a teaspoon of pee, shuffle back to my seat, get comfy and repeat the cycle. Then I couldn't poop for days because of the painkiller. I took many, many stool softeners. When I did finally go, it hurt my stomach so badly that I cried. I never paid attention to how your stomach muscles contract when you "do a two-zie" (pronounced too-zee) as my silly brother would say. It was extremely hot that summer. I sweat a lot in the crease where my stitches were, regardless of what I did to prevent it. The surgical site stayed irritated for a long time. I was so exhausted. It took months until I could walk for exercise again. I got more depressed and experienced mean mood swings. I must have been eating more because I gained more weight, but I wasn't to the point where I paid attention to it.

Finally Got Some Relief

Earlier that year I ended up going to a psychologist, who referred me to a psychiatrist who focused on alternative medicine. This is the doctor I referred to earlier. He had an M.D. as well as a PhD in psychology. For my excessive crying, he prescribed Celexa, which ended up making me feel numb. At least I wasn't crying in the middle of class anymore. He tested my saliva hormone levels and found the low progesterone. He told me about supplementing with natural progesterone cream since it had less side effects than birth control pills. I also have a blood clotting disorder, so I can't take them anyway.

In 2002, I started using the natural progesterone cream. My daily migraines disappeared almost completely! Those migraines were killing me. I couldn't step outside without my sunglasses on. The flashing lights in my eyes distracted me. I never wanted to drive. It was such a relief when they were gone. I felt like my moods swings got better. However, I was taking an antidepressant. It was probably a combo of the two that did the trick. I still couldn't concentrate and had no energy at all. I continued gaining weight and my periods were not regulating.

My sleep cycle got all backwards. I ended up sleeping most days and staying up all night. No matter what I did I couldn't sleep on a regular schedule. I tried sun lamps in the mornings, staying up all night and all day to hopefully pass out at a normal time, moving my bedtime up an hour each day to get it back to a normal time, supplements, etc. Nothing worked until I got a part-time job a couple of years later that I had to get up at 6 a.m. for and HAD to force myself out of bed every day... ok, Chet had to force me out of bed. I didn't feel good in the morning for a couple years.

How Many Doctors is this Now?

Let me take a doctor count up to this point. I saw my family doctor several times, two psychologists, one psychiatrist/alternative medicine doctor, another family doctor and a gynecologist. Nobody up to this point diagnosed me with PCOS. Nobody bothered to test my insulin, which can be high even if your blood sugar is normal, indicating insulin resistance (prediabetes). Nobody tried more than "you have to lose weight". That was a lot of time, money and effort going to all those appointments. "You have to lose weight" ... NO FOOLIN!!!!!!!! I feel like I wasted so much of my time.

By January of 2002 I weighed 333 pounds. I couldn't believe it! I still can't believe it. I bought a treadmill the next day after I weighed myself. I started exercising again that day. I walked slowly for ten minutes, three times a week to start. I was tired. My legs burned and itched like crazy. I think that's called circulation. My knees ached. My butt muscles ached. I was too tired to work. Chet and I were broke. It caused us a lot of problems. We were both extremely anxious all the time.

We skipped bills so we could eat. We ate inexpensive stuff like hot dogs and spaghetti. I felt it was all we could afford. Now I see the irony in it since I somehow found the money to buy my favorite comfort foods. I could have used that money to buy lean meats and produce, but instead I'd buy all this cheap junk food.... cookies, cakes, donuts, chips, ice cream. I would buy cases of candy bars at the wholesale shopper's club. Basically, I skipped bills to buy my favorite drug of choice... junk food.

Didn't Think it Could Get Worse

Nothing seemed to make sense. I was depressed and Chet was depressed. He hated seeing me fall apart. We were not on the same page, yet he was my best friend. My health problems made a lot of problems from his past resurface. I didn't feel like he heard half of what I said. Of course, I wasn't making sense to myself, so it was probably ok that he couldn't hear me.

Chet's depression got severe. He often talked about how it would probably be better if he were dead. He told me repeatedly that he thought about driving into a tree on the way to work to end it. I had never been around someone who seriously wanted to take their own life before. I didn't want to go on in high school some days, but I didn't come close to ending my own life. Something in his tone and the look in his eyes made me feel like he meant it. I was scared and confused as to how to handle the situation.

I told our couple's counselor how Chet had been talking. She suggested I take him to the hospital and have him committed. I knew she was right, but I couldn't believe what I was about to do.

Was he going to give me a hard time? Was I going to have to call for help to take him there? What would I say when I got there?

He did go of his own volition. Deep down I believe he knew it was the best thing for him, but at the time he hated me for it. The twenty-minute drive to the hospital felt like hours. I don't remember talking. The energy in the car was anxious and dark.

It was hard for me to check him in and watch him get stripped of his belongings... they take away anything that may be used for self-harm. I took his shoelaces and his belt home with me. I gave a history to the counselor and then they asked me to leave. I'll never forget the sad, confused look on Chet's face as he looked at me through the glass door that got locked behind me. Depressed and now trapped; somehow, I felt like this could make him worse. People have been watched this way for suicide prevention for years; I had to trust that the professionals knew what they were doing. It was hard for me to watch him go through that, so I cannot imagine how hard it is to go through it yourself... to be that person trapped on the other side of the glass, feeling like you've been deserted by the person who you love the most.

Driving home from the hospital I experienced the loneliest feeling. It was one of the hardest things I've ever done. He was my only family in Virginia. I had nowhere to go but home... back to the big, empty, cold building where I now felt trapped. Both of us feeling alone and trapped. I didn't know what to do with any of this. I didn't want to tell anyone because I didn't want Chet to be embarrassed. The stigma attached to mental health issues runs deep in our society and I didn't want him to be judged. I didn't want people to think differently of him. I didn't want people to think differently of us. I wanted to protect the image I created of Chet and of our relationship.

I didn't sleep that night. I went out and got myself a pack of cigarettes and a bunch of food. I sat on our patio alternating between peanut butter cups, party mix and cigarettes. I woke up with a massive headache. Going from not smoking at all to finishing a whole pack in a night was not a smart move. I couldn't breathe… turns out I also had asthma and didn't know it yet. All I wanted to do was call someone and cry to them. I wanted someone to come stay with me. I needed comfort and support and I didn't know how to ask for it.

Chet was in the hospital for about a week. Then he attended an intensive outpatient program for about a month. He couldn't work that whole time. The doctors were doing their best to get his meds right, but I'm not sure they helped him. All this time I was sad, lonely and confused. I did a good job of isolating myself. I'd have to try hard to keep it light on the phone with whomever I talked to and then I'd hang up and bawl. I remember eating a lot of junk, but I didn't realize at the time that I was attempting to comfort myself with food. I'd beat myself up for being unable to help Chet, then beat myself up about how much I ate and the weight gain. Then I'd go eat some more.

I told Chet I thought we needed a break and I moved into our upstairs bedroom. I concentrated on myself. I needed the space. I didn't feel like he understood anything I told him. I felt like the distance between us was necessary for me to help him too. I didn't want sex to be the answer to fix things. After we would talk it seemed like an argument so we would "makeup". I swear after that he would forget anything I told him. However, he often couldn't focus and forgot a lot I said.

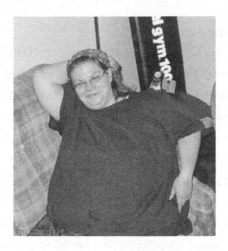

*By the end of 2002 I reached my max weight at close to 350 pounds.
I was 24 years old and feeling completely defeated.*

After looking at Chet's behavior overall, I figured out that he has ADHD and asked him to see a psychiatrist for confirmation. They did the testing and it turned out positive. (Isn't it interesting that most of the time if you have a "positive" test result, it is a bad thing?) I knew he had a sweet heart, so it didn't make sense why he wouldn't listen or remember half of what I said or asked him to do. Did depression issues account for all of it? Was the ADHD impeding his treatment since he literally couldn't concentrate on all he had to do to help himself?

We learned to cope with some of this through lifestyle changes. Again, if you can learn why something is the way it is, you can learn how to deal with it. At any rate, it was better for us to be separated at the time. I was trying to sort out my thoughts and I needed the space to do that. I needed to realize that it was his job to work on himself... I couldn't do the work for him, nor should I have expected myself to do that.

Finally... a Diagnosis!

That spring I did a lot more research on PCOS. I was convinced I had it and set out to find a doctor who would confirm my condition. I found one at Student Health at UVA that Spring. She was a gynecologist. She was very thorough. She listened! She sent me for a bunch of tests to rule out other conditions before making her diagnosis. The tests came back as we both anticipated. Based on them and my physical symptoms she made the diagnosis of PCOS. Oddly enough it brought relief. All my time and energy finally paid off. I felt like a complete mess, mentally and physically, for three years. Now I had direction. I could finally move forward. It'd be best to read a little more about PCOS before we continue my journey

Chapter 4
What is Polycystic Ovary Syndrome (PCOS)?

This book is not intended to be a reference book for Polycystic Ovary Syndrome (PCOS). There are books and websites listed in the Recommended Reading section if you'd like more information. However, I wanted to give a general description of the signs, symptoms and treatment since I mention it quite often.

It is estimated that 5-10% of the female population has PCOS. It is a hormonal disorder that has a huge impact on many aspects of a woman's life. A hormone is a chemical messenger that helps communication between the cells of our bodies. I think of it as if our cells are passing notes to one another to communicate, like most of us did in middle school. They regulate our bodies' functions. Our hormones have to be in balance. They are often likened to a symphony; the instruments must play at the correct times, with the correct notes and volume to produce beautiful music. Similarly, our hormones must be in the proper levels and ratios for our bodies to function optimally. PCOS is one example of what happens when our hormones are not in the proper levels or ratios.

The main hormones imbalanced in patients with PCOS are insulin, estrogen, progesterone, testosterone, LH (luteinizing hormone) and FSH (follicle stimulating hormone), although many others are probably affected as well. These hormones are found in both sexes, but they are in different levels and ratios.

PCOS is characterized by elevated "male" hormones, mainly testosterone, and chronic anovulation, meaning you don't release an egg, or ovulate, during your menstrual cycle. Signs and symptoms, blood work results and a transvaginal ultrasound (an ultrasound taken through the vagina) of the ovaries will help determine a diagnosis of PCOS. It is important for your doctor to rule out other disorders when trying to make a diagnosis because many of the signs and symptoms overlap with other disorders.

The most common signs and symptoms of PCOS are:
- irregular periods with chronic anovulation
- obesity/weight gain
- hyperinsulinemia, insulin resistance, diabetes
- dyslipidemia – high cholesterol and triglycerides
- hirsutism -excessive hair growth, usually on the face, arms and abdomen
- hair loss, male pattern baldness
- miscarriage
- infertility
- depression
- premenstrual syndrome (PMS)
- acne
- acanthosis nigricans - patches of velvety skin with changes in pigmentation, generally found on the back of the neck
- hypertension - high blood pressure

Taken together, insulin resistance, dyslipidemia (specifically decreased HDL and increased triglycerides), hypertension and central obesity (apple shape or "top heavy") leads to a diagnosis of metabolic syndrome. It is common in women with PCOS; however, obesity is a risk factor for this disorder, regardless of PCOS status. It puts a person at a higher risk for type 2 diabetes and cardiovascular disease.

PCOS is often characterized by a low ratio of progesterone to estrogen, and a high ratio of LH to FSH. As the name Polycystic Ovary Syndrome suggests, an ultrasound may show many (poly-) cysts, or a collection of premature follicles (eggs), on the ovaries.

Not all women with PCOS have ovarian cysts. It is important to remember that it is normal to have functional cysts on your ovaries, as they are a part of ovulation. When these cysts cannot develop further and the eggs are not released, they collect on the surface of the ovary, giving it the appearance of a string of pearls.

Most women do not have all the signs and symptoms, often making the diagnosis of PCOS a difficult one. At first glance, many of these symptoms may seem like normal parts of life or are written off as "just running in the family", like having acne, developing facial hair, weight gain and irregular periods. Many women may complain of these symptoms throughout the course of their lives. Unfortunately, many may not think to report all of them at one time. It took me years until I lumped all my problems together and started approaching doctors about them. Even when presented with all my issues, many doctors dismissed me and attributed my concerns to overeating and depression.

Different treatments and combinations of treatments work for some people and not for others. We must listen to our bodies and our hearts. If something works for you, stick with it. If something doesn't work or you don't see any changes, after having given the treatment enough time, discuss stopping that treatment with your doctor. Don't be afraid to speak your mind. A good doctor will listen to your feedback. It is important to realize that we do have options and can give input into our treatment.

The reason I believe not all women have all the symptoms and that some treatments work for some and not others, is because, and I speculate this, but there are probably many hormonal imbalances lumped together and called PCOS. This is why medical professionals call PCO a syndrome. The term "syndrome" refers to a collection of signs and symptoms that often appear together, but do not have a known underlying cause. Thus, it may be that the signs and symptoms overlap for several disease states, awaiting a known cause to be classified as a "disease". As more research is done, more answers will be unveiled. We need to spend more time listening to women and doing more research in women's health. Up until the 1990s many medical research studies excluded women as subjects so they didn't have the added variable of the hormonal fluctuation associated with the menstrual cycle. While scientifically it does make sense to eliminate that pesky fluctuation, it has led to years of discrimination in the medical realm. (Vliet, 2000)

If left untreated, high insulin levels, dyslipidemia, hypertension and estrogen dominance can lead to diabetes, heart disease, some cancers and other disorders. However, many studies have shown that lifestyle modifications can keep our propensities towards some of these diseases in check. Lifestyle changes can make a huge impact on women with PCOS. This is why I found it so overwhelming! Once I got diagnosed, everyone was telling me I needed to eat better and lose weight. I had to do the one thing I hadn't been able to figure out my whole life! I also knew that having high insulin levels made it harder. I felt like the deck was stacked against me. Working on my emotional eating was the best thing I ever did to "treat" my PCOS.

Everything I mention in this book has made me stronger. I continue to learn more things I could be adding or subtracting to help build a healthier body. I don't use any medications to control my symptoms besides the progesterone cream I mentioned in the previous chapter. However, common treatment options include:

- Metformin or other medications to help increase insulin sensitivity and balance out your hormones
- Spironolactone to help reduce the effects of hyperandrogenism
- Cholesterol meds to help with the dyslipidemia
- Birth control to help regulate your cycle (I encourage all

women to learn about the risks of birth control and the
benefits of bio-identical hormone replacement.)

Now that you have an overview of PCOS, you are prepared
to dive forward into the next chapter as I continue my story. The Tilt-
A-Whirl continues….

Chapter 5
Moving Past PCOS

The gynecologist sent me to see an endocrinologist at UVA and he made it sound like my diagnosis was cut and dried. I'm glad it was so easy for "him" to see! Why didn't anyone else know about PCOS?! He prescribed me Metformin to increase my insulin sensitivity and Spironolactone to decrease the effects of the high testosterone levels. I ended up discontinuing the drugs after I tried them for a while, after discussing it with my doctor. I couldn't tolerate the diarrhea and nausea I experienced on the Metformin. I didn't see a difference in the facial hair when I took the Spironolactone. I know some women have positive results with these medications. Everyone's body is different, so not everyone will have the same results.

The endocrinologist sent me to a dietitian. I saw her several times. We talked about the food pyramid, portion control and exercise. I was bored since I knew about this stuff. I still didn't know how to stop eating when I wasn't hungry. She couldn't tell me how to do that. I complained to her about the fact that I got bloated all the time. She ticked me off when she said it was probably coming from my heart's inability to pump efficiently due to my weight. I didn't know she was a dietitian AND a cardiologist!!! How dare she tell me that I had a weak heart? I was in my early twenties and exercised most of my life. Screw her! I never saw her again. Shocking, huh?! She didn't consider the fact that my hormonal imbalance could lead to bloating. Don't most women have times when they get bloated?! I didn't feel bad not going back. It wasn't like I didn't understand that I shouldn't eat a whole box of pasta, but I didn't know how to stop myself. I wasn't ready to acknowledge my food addiction. Plus, it's not like going to a dietitian with a list of foods that I "shouldn't" have eaten would help me stop beating myself up. I didn't need her to tell me that I "should" be eating better or that I "should" be eating less. No foolin'!

My Mom and I attended the PCOSupport conference later that year, which was in Minnesota. PCOSupport is a wonderful support group I found online for women with PCOS. They had great info on their website. I couldn't wait to talk to them in person. I was desperate to get more information; driving from Pennsylvania to Minnesota for the conference didn't seem like a big deal. I got to talk to so many people who knew what I was going through and understood me. There were women there that couldn't lose weight no matter what they did. Women who shaved twice a day instead of once like me. Women who lost a lot of their hair and had to wear wigs. Women who wanted to get pregnant so badly that it consumed them and their spouses. I felt more relaxed there then I had been in years. Relaxed in the middle of all our chaos. Does that make sense? I guess I found peace through their understanding.

Amazing How Much This All Cost

I ended up not being able to do any research while at UVA and I withdrew from the PhD program. I felt like such a failure. This started my panic attacks. My heart would beat like crazy. My palms would sweat. My breathing would become erratic. I would cry. I couldn't go back to the school before I left. I wanted to say goodbye to some of the nice people I had met. I managed to get my Master of Arts in Chemistry from UVA by December 2002, even though I was in a terrible state of mind. I wasn't proud of myself at all. I didn't go to my graduation. One of the main reasons was that I didn't know if the largest gown would fit. All I felt was that I was a failure… once again.

We used all the money that Chet put down on the house as a second mortgage to cover my extensive medical expenses. I ended up needing over $5,000 worth of dental work while we were in VA. I am convinced it was due to my hormones being out of whack. I didn't have health insurance. Chet and I were not married yet and I was over 25 so I couldn't be on my parents' insurance anymore. I saw the alternative medicine/psychiatrist quite a few times at $175 per visit. I spent the money because he was the only one who made sense. He taught me a lot. I was so desperate to feel better that I bought many different supplements and vitamins over the years. I lined them up side by side on our eight-foot kitchen counter once and filled the entire length. I bought stuff to regulate sugar, to block carbs, to speed up metabolism, to help bowel movements, to regulate thyroid, to reduce cortisol, to help me sleep, to boost my immune system, to help with stress, anxiety and depression. I tried them all and none of them worked.

I meditated, prayed, went for counseling, made Chet go with me for counseling, made Chet go for counseling, made him get tested for ADHD, took bubble baths, sang, wrote in my journal, exercised, walked up Skyline Drive to relax (boy, it is beautiful up there), used aroma therapy (the sprays, the under the nose oils, candles), I read books on depression, thyroid, CFS, female health, ADD, immune systems, bowel health and nutrition. I spent an incredible amount of time and money. I didn't know what else to do.

It is amazing when you are ill how fast your money can disappear. I couldn't work for half of time we lived in Virginia, so I lost that income as well. However, I couldn't qualify for any medical assistance or food stamps because our combined income was over a certain amount. As a result, we went over $80,000 in debt.

This experience cost me more than money. The entire time I lived in Virginia I stopped talking to my friends and tried not to let my family know exactly how bad I felt. The more persistent ones kept calling over and over, but I never talked about what was really on my mind. I tried to keep it light. You know… "How's the weather? See any good movies?" Blah, blah, blah. I'd hang up and cry my eyes out. I didn't know what to do with myself. I was restless all the time. I was tired. How could I talk to anyone when all I wanted to do was cry? What could they have done about it? **I realize now that one major way to heal is to talk about how you feel and accept compassion from your loved ones.** (I added this line years after I originally wrote this.)

One of my girlfriends whom I knew since we were little finally wrote me a letter. She asked me what the heck was wrong with me and filled me in on all I missed in her life over the couple years we didn't talk. I'm glad she did. It helped me start looking at what I had done. How did someone who always said her friends and family were a priority completely withdraw from them? How could I let all this fester inside me without letting any of it out? Without asking anyone for help? Sad thing is that many people that suffer from depression end up isolating themselves, which makes it even worse. Unfortunately, many people are uncomfortable talking about their feelings. Many learn to ignore their feelings completely for fear of being broken by them. I was definitely one of those people.

It has been said that our emotions, and our capability of having empathy are what separate us from the animals. I have cats and I don't think that's true. I think they definitely express emotions. They express being angry or scared by hissing, contentment or happiness by purring, or love by cuddling to name a few. However, what does separate us from them is our ability to verbalize our feelings, yet many of us choose not to talk. Strange. We have a thought and a feeling, we can then say it aloud. Why is that hard for so many of us?

Trying to Lose Weight Again… and Get Married?!

I spent that next year, May 2002 to May 2003, trying to lose weight. I swore up and down that I took the Metformin as prescribed and ate what I believed to be healthy, but my weight changed very little. However, I was in better physical shape. I started to work part time at a bookstore. As I said, I found it extremely difficult to get there by 7 a.m., but at least I was doing it. I was on my feet and doing more than I had done for quite some time. I knew I had to be burning more calories. Where was I going wrong?

I kept track of my weight closely and looked for a pattern. I finally realized what happened. Every time I went to visit my family in Scranton or friends in Philly I would gain five pounds. It would take five weeks at home to lose what I gained; a week later I would go back for another visit, gain again, and repeat the cycle. I did this for a whole year. I told my endocrinologist this and he told me about a research study on PCOS and weight loss strategies they were doing. It sounded like a great opportunity. I signed up immediately.

Chet worked on his depression issues and I worked on my own health. We started to reconnect again. The time I spent living upstairs made me realize I didn't want to be without him. We continued to go for counseling. I felt that if we could get through all this stuff we were meant to be together. I re-proposed to him since I'm the one who originally called it off, and we got married a few months later.

Our wedding was perfect with one huge exception. We got married at a time when I felt disconnected to people I loved. I managed to get most of my girlfriends together, but I had stopped talking to most of my guy friends. I think it was partly because my problems were "female" and I wouldn't have wanted to bother them with my period or mood problems. I realize now they probably wouldn't have minded if I cried to them either. I've always been surrounded by loving, supportive people and for that I am truly grateful. I managed to push many of them away over the years, and for that I am truly sorry.

We had an outdoor ceremony at McDade Park in Scranton, one of my old favorite running spots, and a cookout afterwards. It wasn't what we had originally planned back in August 2001, but I think it was better. I think that often when young couples get married they don't know what their vows mean. We knew exactly what they meant. We lived together and supported each other in sickness and health, richer and very poorer, good times and very bad. We knew we would be good at it. We both bawled. I was surprised to see that reaction from Chet... I'd only seen him cry a few times. That was the most emotion I felt at one time and I am sure it was the same for him. We were blessed to have found one another. We helped each other through a lot over the years.

Emotional Eating?

After our wedding, I jumped right into the research study. The lifestyle coach asked me to keep a food journal. We examined the patterns together. We ended up talking a lot about emotional eating. I started reading as much as I could about it. The names of some of the books can be found at the back of this book in the Recommended Reading section. They hit home. They talked about food in a way that I had never heard before. It was quite overwhelming.

I lost weight and exercised a lot more being in the research study. I appreciated having the accountability. Having someone to report to every week helped keep me on track. I think our weekly visits helped more than the Metformin. I went off the Celexa, partly because I felt better, and partly because I couldn't afford it anymore.

I was improving, but we couldn't stay in Virginia. The money ran dry. Every day we stayed was one more step we were taking further into debt. I wouldn't be returning to school any time soon and we couldn't afford our house, second mortgage payments and credit card payments anymore. I still didn't feel like I had the energy to work full-time. If I did continue to work at the bookstore, my salary wouldn't have helped that much anyway.

Moving Back Home

We left our jobs in Virginia in December 2003. We had one week to get packed before we brought our first truck up to the house. We moved back into Chet's house in Wilkes-Barre, PA. We were extremely busy. We packed, cleaned, fixed up anything in our house in VA that needed fixing, painted and unpacked again. Did I mention that neither of us had jobs at that point yet?

Chet decided to go back to college when we moved back home. He was 25 years older than most of his fellow students. I was proud of him for taking that step. I knew he wanted to do it for a while, and I thought it would help keep him out of his depression. He had been supportive of me in Virginia and I felt like it was my turn to support him. He deserved to be happy and feel productive. It was a big gamble but it worked. Chet graduated May 2006 with an Associate Degree in Electrical Engineering. He found a position working as a broadcast engineer and he fell in love with it. I'm happy that he could concentrate on himself and reach his goals. He became happier and felt more productive than he had in years. Our relationship got stronger as a result. We were finally both moving forward in what seemed to be the same direction.

I started working in the Admissions Department at a hospital conveniently located less than a mile from our house by the end of February 2004. I was thrilled to work in the hospital; I spent a lot of time in one over the years and I felt at home. Also, I knew how crappy you feel when you are sick and I wanted to help people out. I wanted to make them smile. I still do. It's amazing how much you can affect someone's mood with kindness.

I was awfully tired when I started back to work. The first thing I would do when the alarm went off was curse. "Shit!" I seriously couldn't believe eight hours passed!!! I never felt rested. Half the time I didn't hear the alarm and Chet had to wake me up. Many mornings I wanted to cry. I did cry.

It took time to get settled in Wilkes-Barre and adjust to working full-time again. I think it took about a year, but then I started doing more research on food addiction and emotional eating. That is when I started the journal that has become this book. Making major shifts in my thinking was quite the process. In the following chapters I share my struggles and my victories along the way.

First Steps

Now you know a lot about me. It's time to learn about you. First, I review some of the reasons people eat and common thinking traps. The next couple of chapters will help you take a closer look at your own relationship with food. It may be difficult to look at yourself, but it will be the best decision you've ever made. You can do it. Keep reading and stay open-minded. If you're curious to see where my life has gone, I catch you up to date with more of my story later in the book.

When you start out on any journey it can look daunting. Do yourself a favor... next time you are headed up a big hill, notice how far away the top appears, then look down at the next few feet. Moving forward doesn't seem difficult at that point, when all you can see are the next few steps and you can barely tell you are facing up a hill. All you need to do is keep moving one foot in front of the other and keep going. You'll get to the top before you know it, and you'll be looking for the next hill you'd like to climb!

Chapter 6
Lies, Traps & Excuses

When it comes to weight loss, food rules, and body image we've all been subjected to common lies and traps. The lies may start as something someone once told you or something you heard through the media. Eventually they became commonplace in your mind and the lies become your "truths". Thoughts like:

I can't do this.

I'm weak.

I'm lazy.

I'll never be thin, so why bother trying.

I'm a failure.

You can't eat that, you're too fat.

I screwed it up so why not continue "being bad" for the rest of the day... week... etc.

I am "less than" because I do not fit into the mold of what "people" consider beautiful.

It is all garbage, but many of us fixate on these thoughts throughout the day. It may seem normal to you because you've always done it. It seemed normal to me to have this background tape of negativity playing in my mind. I thought I should be thinking that way since I had weight to lose. I somehow felt I deserved to berate myself. I failed over and over so I should be punished... and I did punish myself every single day for years. I let my mind beat me up.

Many of these negative thoughts probably leave your mouth. Self-degradation has become common in our society and is often ignored. Have you been out with friends and someone starts the self-bashing? I hate my _____ (fill in the blank with whatever body part you like… dimply thighs, jiggly stomach, fat butt, etc.). People often take turns in the group until everyone has named something about themselves that they hate. By the time it's done the whole energy of the group has shifted to the negative. It can be contagious. We have to make a conscious effort to stop our negative thoughts and help those around us stop as well. We need to be a lot nicer to ourselves, and to each other….

Sizism… Can't We All be Nice?

What if weight were proportionate to how bad people felt? Would people think that fat is funny then? Our society continues to allow sizism to occur; it is sad that negativity often unifies us. Fat can be picked on by anyone, regardless of race, religion, socioeconomic status, and even size! For some reason people who are overweight or obese feel that they can pick on others for their weight. This makes no sense! Over 70% of Americans are overweight or obese, so why are we picking on each other?! Why don't we join together and stop it from happening?

There is an application on smartphones where you can take a picture of people and change their face into a fatter version of themselves. This is appalling! At first glance, maybe it seems amusing to take thin people, or maybe actors or actresses who are thin, and transform them to be fat. But what if the fat on their body were proportionate to their pain, either the pain they currently feel, or past pains? What if the number of donuts consumed to get that big were equal to the sense of loss and emptiness they felt when losing a son or daughter, or because they couldn't deal with the chronic pain they felt after being in an accident? And, if you were to take a picture of my face now and perform this application on it, I would look like I looked years ago… when I was overcome with sadness and an overwhelming feeling of loss of motivation and control. This is not funny. Fat isn't funny.

Let's stop making it ok to pick on fat. Let's make the conscious effort to be nicer to ourselves, to stick up for ourselves and other people, and start using more positive language in general. Let's be nice people!

And let's start being honest with ourselves...

The "But I Don't Eat that Much" Lie

I think this is one of the hardest ones to face. I don't know how many times I told myself and other people in my life that one. I have had patients who are carrying hundreds of extra pounds stare right into my eyes and swear that they don't eat that much. I think we don't want to believe that we overeat because we don't think we can change it. We don't want to believe our weight gain is our fault. I used to eat a lot more than I thought I did. Part of the problem is that we don't pay enough attention to what goes into our mouths. If you believe this one please don't be offended. Instead be brave and take a good hard look at what you are doing with food. You are probably eating more than you think. Maybe you are not, but I encourage you to take a good look to be certain.

The Night Eating Trap

This one goes hand in hand with **The I Should Skip Breakfast Trap.** Many people I've talked to have fallen into the night eating trap. I did it for a long time. I'd wake up feeling like I ate too much the day before. Maybe I'd weigh myself for confirmation... to make myself feel worse for eating at night so I wouldn't do it again. Then I'd either skip breakfast completely or have a small piece of fruit. Then I'd keep using my 'willpower' to get me through lunch, have something light, skip my snack and wait until I'd get home for dinner. Well, by the time dinner rolled around I'd be super hungry. I'd snack while I prepared dinner. Then I'd eat a bigger portion of food than normal. Then I'd eat dessert... I might as well since *'I hadn't eaten much during the day'*. Then, sitting around in front of the television or computer I'd snack since **'I hadn't eaten much during the day'** so I deserved to snack. I'd eat way more than my body needed for fuel. Then I'd eat more because I had **'already blown it'** for the day.

I've awakened in the middle of the night to eat. I'd go periods of depriving myself of food, then wake up feeling extremely hungry and eat a whole bunch of food. This was usually during times of high stress. I've stayed up through the night to graze as well. I wouldn't necessarily binge on a lot of food at one time, but I'd keep a steady, slow snack pace all through the night. For example, I may not eat a whole cake in a half hour, but I'd eat a slice every hour.

A lot of night eating has nothing to do with physical hunger. At night, we are often left alone with our thoughts... our feelings can creep in and start to disturb us. We reach for food to avoid thinking about the things that are bothering us. I had to convince myself that I was not physically hungry at night... that food was not going to fix whatever was going on. I often reached for food shortly after eating dinner, so I knew it was not physical hunger. I kept reminding myself that I had to dig a little deeper to see what was bothering me. If nothing was wrong, I had to remind myself that I was eating out of habit and I had to break it. I started figuring out how to soothe myself at night. As I would journal or talk to a friend, I would have a warm cup of herbal tea. The warmth of the tea was comforting. I had that habitual hand to mouth action, but consumed less calories in the process.

One of the most important things you can do to help get out of this trap is to start eating breakfast, even if you are not hungry when you get up. I know, I know... this seems opposite of what you "should" do. Why would you eat when you are not hungry? It feels like you will eat more food throughout the day, and you are trying to eat less. I want you to become more mindful of your physical hunger. However, your body's metabolic clock is probably messed up if you are falling into a pattern when you eat more at night and skip breakfast. You can help get out of it by eating breakfast within an hour or so of waking to help reset your meal patterns and stop the cycle of overeating at night. Eat something for breakfast, then focus the rest of the day on eating when you are physically hungry and stopping when you are satisfied. This is the foundation of mindful eating. I'll challenge you to think more about physical hunger and satisfaction in later chapters.

The "I'll Start Again Monday" Trap

'I'll start again Monday.' How many times have you told yourself that? I screwed up so much today, that I might as well start again next week. This line of thinking can occur regardless of what day it is… it could even be Monday and you'd be looking to start over the following week. That one slip-up, or episode of *'blowing it'* as many of us call it, leads to this feeling of self-loathing and regret. It leads to the feeling that you might as well continue to mess it up since you had *'gone off your diet'* anyway. It can turn into a week of beating yourself up, feeling guilty and eating more and more while you wait for that next Monday to come.

Try thinking about each moment as if it were a new "Monday". This Tuesday when you find yourself overeating, think to yourself that this moment of *'blowing it'* is over and you can start over again right this very minute. Your second, fourteenth or 5,000th chance doesn't have to wait until the next time it says Monday on the calendar. "Monday" can be right now. It can be after you ate dessert when you knew you were full. It can be after that mid-afternoon snack at work that you ate only to be social. That mid-afternoon candy bar on a Wednesday doesn't have to be the spark that leads to the toilet bowl thinking of failure that makes you not want to try to build a healthier relationship with food until the following Monday. Practicing new behaviors can start right now, in the present moment. With mindful eating every moment is "Monday".

Again, what you will be working on is not a "diet"... it is building a healthy relationship with food. However, you may find yourself beating yourself up during the process too. You can push the date forward when you will make the effort to be mindful of your eating, like starting over on Monday, OR you can start becoming self-aware right now. Part of healing is knowing that it is a process. Accept that your behaviors will not change overnight. You will know as you are doing something that it is the very behavior you wish to stop, but you are not able to at that moment.... yet. Give yourself a break. Stop judging yourself.

The Last Supper Trap

If you stop the '**I'll Start Again Monday**' trap, you will help yourself avoid the '**Last Supper**' trap. You know that feeling that you get when you know you are about to start a diet. The '*boy, I'd better eat all these things that I know I will have to restrict*' feeling. I had better eat this cake tonight since it'll be a while until I can have any cake again. I had better go to my favorite restaurant a few times this week for that chicken Alfredo, since I know I shouldn't be eating that on my new diet. I had better finish all these leftovers this week because none of these foods fit into my new diet plan. I had better finish off the junk food in the house since I'm not going to waste it and throw it out. How many times have you had a Last Supper?

If you are allowing yourself to eat whatever you like... whatever you are craving... there is no need for a Last Supper or kitchen "clean-up". There will be no foods that are necessarily off limits as long as you are eating them when you are physically hungry and stopping when you are satisfied, not stuffed. When start to focus on how your body feels when you eat certain foods you will not eat the same foods in the same quantities. It will take time to figure out how your body responds to certain foods, but if you keep removing those foods from your house that you have deemed "bad", you'll never figure out if your body feels ok when you eat them. I promise you, your cravings will change over time. You won't be compelled to eat a huge piece of cake after dinner. One day you'll crave fruit instead. Another day you will realize you are perfectly content with how you feel after eating dinner and you'll skip dessert, even if it is right in front of you. I never, ever would have imagined that would be the case, but I promise you it does happen!

The "I Won't be Happy Until I'm ___ pounds" Trap

Many of us don't live our lives the way we want to because we let our weight hold us back. For years I thought I had to get to under 200 pounds until I could allow myself to be happy. I had to wait to buy that dress I wanted… to wait to get that new perfume…. to dance in front of people… to go to the beach in my swimsuit… to start dating. I couldn't allow myself to feel pretty, or certainly not sexy, until I hit that magic weight. All these years later and I have never been less than 200 pounds. I would still be waiting to be happy.

You can find happy at any weight. You can start doing more today, regardless of your weight. It may be something that seems simple to other folks. Maybe you've wanted to wear a sleeveless shirt even though you have a history of hating your chubby arms. You can go sleeveless right now. The thought of it may stir up quite a bit of panic. It probably won't feel good the first time you do it, but you'll get used to it. You'll eventually feel that it's not a big deal. Then you may go a step further and do something crazy like wear a swimsuit in public! The sky's the limit folks!

The "Being Heavy Runs in My Family so There Probably Isn't Anything I Can do About it" Trap

Many people have told me that one. Yes, our makeup is largely determined by our genetics. Yes, you may be pre-programmed to be a bigger person. However, a lot of the undesirable behaviors you learned from your family, or from the people in your immediate environment, you can unlearn by teaching yourself new ones. While it is true that I will never be a size 6 with a flat tummy, it doesn't mean that I can't work on my self-image, thought processes and fitness to become the best version of me that I can become. You don't have to put limits on yourself. Stop defeating yourself before you try!

The I'm Good or Bad Depending on If I Eat "Good" or "Bad" Foods Trap

How many times have you heard yourself or someone else say *"I was good today, I didn't eat that _____"*; or *"I was bad today, I had _____ for lunch"*. Our language indicates that there is moral value attached to our food. No wonder we feel so darn guilty about what we put in our mouth!

It's not surprising that it confuses us. Have you noticed that your good and bad food list has changed over the years? If you were on a low-fat diet, you were "good" if you ate fruit, but "bad" if you ate nuts. If you were on a low-carb diet, you were "bad" if you ate fruit, but "good" if you ate nuts. If you were eating low-calorie foods only, you were "good" if you ate fruit, and "bad" if you ate nuts. If you were on the high-fiber diet, you were probably "good" if you ate both fruit and nuts. If you were on a popular weight-loss plan that considered fruit "free", then if you ate fruit you were probably "good" ... "free" would imply good, don't you think? Who can keep it all straight?!! It's maddening! No wonder we are mixed up!!! **Did you notice how none of those diets had anything to do with eating when you are physically hungry?**

Instead of paying attention to some list of approved foods, we should learn to take cues from our bodies. It will tell us what is good for it if we pay attention. If your tummy doesn't bother you when you eat certain foods and if you have energy afterwards, that would be good. Clients tell me they avoid certain foods because they bother their stomach. Does one small cheeseburger bother your stomach, or does it bother you when you eat a double quarter-pound cheeseburger? Often our body reacts negatively when we eat too much. Eating smaller quantities of my favorite foods often leaves me feeling fine. I encourage you to start to challenge your idea of what a "good" food means.

Along with The Traps goes The Excuses

Quit it with the excuses. The excuses are another form of lies you've been telling yourself. I've said them all myself and I've heard them all. Stop letting them get in your way!

I don't have time.

I'm too busy with my family.

I'm too busy at work.

I'm a student and I can't fit it all in.

I'm broke. I can't afford the gym, to see a counselor or a dietitian.

I'm too tired.

I get too sore when I work out.

I can't go very fast when I walk, so there is no point.

You haven't lived my life… it's been too hard.

I'm afraid it won't stick.

The list goes on and on. What have been your excuses? What is stopping you from taking the time to focus on you?

Nobody can do the work for you. I know many of us are caregivers, whether we are parents or not. I know you've heard it before, but it's true... unless you take care of yourself, you won't be able to take care of others to the best of your ability. That's why when you're on a plane that's going down you should put your oxygen on first.... you must continue breathing yourself so you can help others that need you. If you practice caring for yourself, you will be stronger and have more energy to help your loved ones.

Decide to stop. Stop doubting yourself. Stop feeling like you are not worth the effort. Stop complaining. Stop beating yourself up. Catch yourself when you are making excuses in your mind and tell yourself to stop.

Every day you have the choice to fight for yourself or give in to old habits. You can choose to do things to make you a better version of you, or you can do nothing and feel bad about it and yourself. Decide that you are worth the effort. Fight for yourself. Nobody can do it for you. If you start fighting you may find it's contagious. You may find that there are others in your life who not only want to help you, but who want to fight for themselves as well.

The Enabler Trap

A lot of people think they can't work on their food issues in the environment they are in. When I was younger, I would blame my family. I was around people who snacked a lot, so I snacked a lot. I used to think that my weight had a lot to do with my husband's food habits too. He'd have chips, cookies, soda, cakes, and donuts in the house. I didn't think I could be around that stuff. If he didn't have it in the house I couldn't eat it, right? In theory that is the case, but we are always around food. Every day we are surrounded by that which tempts us. If you heal your relationship with food, it won't tempt you nearly as often. You will be able to be in a house that has cookies, soda, cakes, chips and donuts and not think about them. You won't consume them unless you are physically hungry and want to eat those things. Eventually you'll want to eat them less often than you think. There are many days now when I choose a piece of fruit over a cookie or some chips. I have learned that fruit makes my body feel better. I know right now you may think the likelihood of that happening is about the same as you seeing a unicorn on your front lawn. I felt that way too. Believe it… I'm telling you it can happen. You are the only one who can heal your relationship with food and with yourself. Stop blaming other people for their supposed sabotage.

The Don't Cry Trap

It is not only food-related traps that we fall into. Some of the traps have to do with feelings and expressing them. "Don't cry" for example… How many times have you heard that? Don't cry. Crying makes those around you uncomfortable. It can make the people who love you feel sad with you and for you. This is unpleasant. In general, we all like to avoid unpleasant stuff. "Don't cry" can be a knee-jerk reaction. I can't tell you how many times I've heard someone tell me that.

A nurse told one of my patients not to cry today. This patient has a chronic infection in her leg, is in danger of losing her leg, is over five hundred pounds and is having trouble paying for her healthcare. She hasn't been able to walk for almost six months. She relies on people around her to do everything for her. She feels like a burden. She feels helpless. She finally admitted to herself and to me that she uses food to cope with her life. If she doesn't deserve a good cry, then who the heck does?! I say cry it out sister!!!

In a way, I'm pleased when I see people cry. Crying is a release. I see it as a way for sadness, stress and many other emotions to escape… to leave us. If we don't feel the feelings we are having and eventually release them, they will fester up inside us. We then try to squash our feelings with food… or other things we may be addicted to, because we cannot stand how they live inside us and eat us up.

Crying connects our body and mind/emotions. By telling ourselves we cannot cry we are starting the disconnect. Allowing yourself to cry is allowing your body to connect to your mind/heart. Learning to identify your feelings, process them, and deal with them in a healthy way is an important step to take in healing yourself.

The "I Can Never Say No Because I Can't Let People Down or They Won't Love Me" Trap

Goes hand in hand with…

The "I Have to Be Strong for Everyone Else because They Expect Me to be, so I Can't Lean on Them" Trap

A lot of my clients have admitted that they are the ones in the family or circle of friends who gets leaned on… they are not the leaners. They have built themselves up as the one who is strong, who can take all the crap that their friends and family throws at them, but who never gets to throw any of their crap back. They end up seeing everyone around them as fragile… as needing protection. They end up feeling that their loved ones need protection from them as well.

I know I felt this way for a long time. I felt like a burden last year with a disabling health issue that went on for the better part of the year. In the past I would have put on a brave face for everyone, regardless of how I felt. I'd keep it up in front of people, but the minute I was alone I'd bawl my eyes out. I wouldn't want anyone to know how bad I felt. I wouldn't want to appear weak. I didn't want them to worry about me. I didn't want people to see me as fragile… being strong for everyone else was a big part of my identity. I was the Protector. I was The Strong One. If I started being real in front of everyone and admitted that I was feeling weak, then who was I?

What would I use to define me? One of the biggest ways I coped with my issues that year was to talk about it. I cried to people and accepted their comfort, hugs and tissues. It made the whole situation much more tolerable, and I didn't turn to food. Nobody accused me of being weak. Nobody needed protection from me and my feelings.

If that has been your pattern it can take a while to break out of it. You can start working on the relationships you have with people a little at a time. It will feel odd at first, like with anything new, but you'll get used to it. You'll end up feeling closer to your loved ones when you share the real parts of you.

Can our feelings break us?

Deep down some of us feel like our feelings will break us. That is a lie too. Sometimes you can simply sit and be with your feelings. We are often desperate to do something about bad feelings. We don't want to feel unpleasant things. Food will never fix whatever it is you are trying to fix. There are many things you can try to do to feel better, but sometimes you will go through something that you need to feel bad about until you don't feel as bad anymore. I know that is a vague statement. We all would like to know when the hurt and pain will end, but you can never predict how long it will take. You have to remind yourself that your feelings will not break you. One of my friends would disagree with me. She thinks she has seen me "broken" at least twice from two different sets of horrible circumstances. Even if she is right, after I "broke" I grew as a person, redefined who I am, and set new goals for myself and came out better for it in the end. It reminds me of a broken bone... sometimes doctors need to break it to reset it correctly before it can mend itself, making it stronger than before.

When my Gram passed away it tore me apart. She was one of my best friends, my cheerleader and my sense of stability. She grounded me. I cried every day for about three months. At first I cried several times per day, then it dwindled down to one time. I would go about my day as usual, but during my ride home from school I would bawl. I had to get the hurt out of my system. I don't know if that's excessive or not. All I knew was that I hurt and had to process it. It took as long as it took. Peanut butter cups were not going to help that pain release any faster. I was in a highly stressful situation mourning her while trying to help my husband with his depression, teach college courses, and keep up with my own school work. Crying helped me release all of that. You can do as many positive things to cope as you can, but sometimes you need to feel bad until you don't.

A lot of the time it is our own negative thoughts making us feel bad. The good news is that you are the one who chooses your thoughts. You can shift your thinking to the positive. It will take time, especially if this type of negative thinking has been happening for years, but you can train yourself to stop. Without viewing yourself through this negative lens you'll be amazed at how differently you can experience life.

Can you think of any lies and traps you've succumbed to that I haven't highlighted? Are you going to keep letting them hold you back?

Chapter 7
Why are You Eating?

When I was bigger many people would offer advice on how to get smaller. I'd hear a lot about what foods to eat, what foods to avoid, how much to eat and how to cook the food. All this focus on *what* and *how*, but nobody asked me *why* I was eating. I want to ask you, "Why are you eating? Are you hungry, or do you want food?" These are often two different things.

Emotional eating, food addiction and mindless eating are concepts that are not new, but they are considered socially acceptable to a point. Many of us have come to accept that it is "just the way it is." It is all around us and has become part of our culture. In fact, I was watching a TV program that showed someone who lost a race for local office sitting alone in a dark room, clearly upset for his loss, spraying whipped cream out of a can right into his mouth. A young woman broke up with her boyfriend on another show and her mom told her part of the healing process was to wallow, watch movies all weekend in her pajamas, and eat as much pizza and ice cream as she wanted. She went a step further and brought out a half gallon of ice cream, two spoons, and sat next to her to help her with the process. As if the ice cream was going to make her feel better! It never does. A character on yet a different show said he knew exactly what flavor pie would go along with his disappointment. Flip through the channels or look around you... people are always trying to use food to make them feel better.

"Why would I do drugs, when I could do veal parmesan?"
-Uncle Joe
Exactly the point Uncle Joe. Many of us think that way!

Physical Hunger versus Emotional Hunger

A lot of us eat when we are not physically hungry. Until I started practicing eating when I was hungry, I never paid attention to physical hunger. I didn't even know what it felt like. I grazed all day, so I never experienced a growling stomach. That's the biggest sign that our body gives that it needs energy. If you are physically hungry, your body needs that fuel to burn. Regardless of the food you choose to eat, your body will burn more than it will store when you are truly physically hungry. That's how the chemistry in our body works. This concept helped take away a lot of the guilt I associated with food. As far as energy is concerned, the body does not care if the sugar comes from fruit, milk, white bread, peanut butter cups, etc. ... the glucose goes through all the same reactions to give us energy. Physical hunger is the main sign that our body needs more glucose to go through those reactions.

Most of us have a lot of stress to process. People in general struggle with similar issues. Instead of talking about it or trying to process it, many of us hold all the stress and bad feelings inside. Then we try to cover it up with food. That is emotional hunger. Many people reach for salty or sugary snacks for a pick-me-up. I have learned which foods I typically reach for when I am sad or stressed, which gives me a clue I am looking to fill an emotional need. Emotional hunger often feels like a void or a longing for something.

Physical hunger comes on slowly if you pay attention to it. You won't get this sudden urge to eat something, like you do when you are emotionally triggered to eat. For example, say I get off the phone with my brother with whom I argued and I want to reach for peanut butter cups. That urgent feeling of "needing" peanut butter cups is an emotional hunger. In that moment, I am trying to soothe myself. Peanut butter cups won't fix the fact that he hurt my feelings. If I stop myself and think about my desire for the peanut butter cups, I can ask myself if I am physically hungry... if my body is telling me I need fuel. If my stomach isn't growling, I don't feel like I have low energy, I don't have a headache or I'm not especially spacy-headed, I know I am not physically hungry.

Another way you can learn to distinguish between physical hunger and emotional hunger is noticing when you are satisfied. True physical hunger can be satisfied with a small amount of food. A midmorning yogurt can hold you over until lunch. A rumbling tummy in the afternoon can be quenched with a handful of almonds until dinner. Emotional hunger doesn't get satisfied by the food because food won't fix the emotional need. For example, you may find yourself sitting on your couch late at night wondering how you find yourself in a situation you are in, while eating ice cream. That ice cream won't fix the fact that you are getting divorced, have a sick family member or financial difficulties. The emotional need you have for support, understanding and reassurance won't be found in the bottom of that ice cream bowl or the bottom of that half gallon container. Regardless of how much you eat, you won't be satisfied.

Food Addiction

The word addiction means different things to different people. When I first thought of addiction, I thought of people in rehab for drug or alcohol abuse. I envisioned the afflicted, shaking in the corner of their substance-free bedroom, coming down from a lifelong high. Then I started to realize that addiction could be subtler, yet no less painful. The substance didn't have to be a "substance". People can be addicted to the feeling certain activities give them. For example, you can have addictions to shopping, shoplifting, gambling, extreme sports, exercising or sex. All addictions produce or numb a feeling. Food did that for me for a long time.

A simple definition of addiction is "an attempt to control the uncontrollable in our lives in the search for happiness." (Nakken,

1996) It is trying to find intimacy through an event or object. Events or objects are more reliable than people: a person with an addiction can count on abusing a substance or partaking in a ritual. For example, the TV never disagrees with you, your beer calms you down and your desserts will never reject you. You forget your pain while you search for your next hit of a drug, sex partner, purchase, sure bet or cheeseburger. The search gives you the feeling that you have control over your life. The high helps you forget your pain.

After you have used that substance or partaken in your addictive activity of choice, you lose that high, pseudo-relaxed feeling. You return to reality feeling worse than before you started since that high and false sense of control is gone. The cycle repeats itself, the whole time the addiction grows stronger. You start to hide your behavior so your loved ones don't think there is anything wrong. Before you know it, you are shutting out your loved ones and withdrawing more into yourself. You don't share how you feel and you keep indulging in your addictive behavior to cope. Before long you lose touch with yourself and your own emotions. You try to fight the addict within, but he/she takes over.

Addiction is tricky. As a way to continue living inside you, the addict knows he/she can change the object of addiction. You may switch back and forth between food, alcohol, gambling, or any other substance or event, giving the appearance that you dealt with your issues. For example, I met a young woman who had been anorexic, who became a binge eater, who turned to excessive exercise and then to smoking and shopping. She didn't deal with her underlying issues, so she continued looking for happiness through many different objects of addiction. When you do this, you end up with low self-esteem, feeling like there is no way out. It is the same process for all addictions. Therefore, the healing process is similar. It is not surprising that an organization like Overeaters Anonymous exists, which is similar to programs for people who suffer from various addictions, like alcohol, drugs or gambling. Since addiction is essentially an unhealthy relationship with an object, you need to "break up" with that object and make sure you don't turn to another one. You need to make serious shifts in your internal dialogue, your relationship with yourself and with the people in your life.

Some people don't understand the concept of a food addiction. It is hard to understand how something we physically need every day can be addicting. We need food to sustain life. It is too easy to blame people for carrying excess weight, feeling like it is their fault because they have no self-control; there is more to it than eating less and moving more. If it were that easy, we'd all be at a healthy weight. Most of us are overweight or obese, so we are surrounded by people who have similar struggles.

There is a physical and emotional component to all addictions. People use drugs because the drug itself produces a euphoric feeling. The drug keeps your brain chemicals in a state where you feel good, giving rise to the physical addiction. Food addiction is no different. Many of the foods people choose to binge on temporarily create a change in your brain chemistry, giving you a short-lived sense of "happiness". Those high-fat, high-sugar snacks temporarily elevate serotonin and dopamine (Barry, Clarke, & Petry, 2009). Certain individuals may be more susceptible to rises in those brain chemicals, essentially being wired for food addiction. That predisposition does not mean that it cannot be controlled in time. That physical component is a lot to overcome, even if you do not have emotional reasons for your addiction in the first place. However, many people develop addictions to escape from how they feel. Not being able to cope with life's struggles or a low self-esteem is the emotional component of addiction.

It is a viscous cycle: the more you reach for food to cheer you up, the more weight you will gain. Being overweight often leads to a low self-esteem. Low self-esteem often leads to depression. Then you need a pick-me-up and guess what follows…you end up reaching for food. The cycle repeats; hence, the addiction begins and grows stronger.

Some people eat because something upsets them. Then they end up feeling bad about themselves for eating. That "feeling bad about themselves" part gets familiar and comfortable. It ends up being easier to feel that self-loathing, rather than to feel the original feeling that made them eat in the first place. For example, it was easier for me to beat myself up about overeating, than to feel like a failure about not continuing towards a doctorate degree. So, I'd feel bad about school, eat something, get the initial rush, crash, and settle into that old familiar habit of feeling bad about being fat, instead of feeling bad about not finishing school. That is what happens when you don't learn to express yourself or get help from others. Here is the lousy part: you eventually end up reaching for food without realizing why you're doing it. It's not like I sat around thinking, "Gee, I feel like crap about not getting my PhD, so I am going to sit here and shove my face." All I knew was that I felt hungry. Hungry for me equaled happy, sad, mad, frustrated, depressed, anxious, disgusted, lonely or scared. I didn't end up paying attention to my emotions; I knew I was "hungry". Most of it was emotional hunger.

Mindless Eating

You may not recognize yourself as an emotional eater or a food addict. Maybe you don't feel like you have a stressful life and that you have no emotional triggers that cause you to eat. Another answer to "Why are you eating?" may simply be "I have no idea!" It may be that you are not paying attention. It may be that you have been trained to eat at certain times, in specific places, or around certain people and don't give it much thought. How many times have you walked by a candy dish and grabbed a handful when you weren't hungry? It's amazing how often we do that without realizing it. How many times have you eaten a snack in the car, on the couch or at the movies because you *always* do? Eating is often a habit, an automatic response.

We are all extremely busy these days. We barely pay attention to many things we do. We are so used to multi-tasking and running on autopilot that this type of zoning out also applies to eating. How many times have you opened a bag of chips, got distracted by TV, internet, or family, finally look in the bag again, and most of them or all of them were gone? Where did those darn chips go?! Many people get another snack since they missed the experience of eating the first snack. You may have a second dessert because you barely tasted the first one. Some people do this at most meals or snack times. At one point, I know I did. This can add up to an incredible number of calories throughout the day.

In my experience, men do not as freely admit to emotional or stress-eating as women. In general, men have been taught to be "the strong ones". Many are taught they are not allowed to cry or show emotion. If they do, they may have experienced being called names, and often could have been likened to a female, which for some reason makes them feel weak. The phrase "emotional eating" to some may imply weakness. Admitting to stress-eating would imply that they could not deal with their stress… not very "masculine", right? Personally, I think that is ridiculous since all human beings have feelings and likely have been overwhelmed by them on occasion. Women may be more emotional creatures, but that doesn't mean that men should prevent themselves from admitting to these behaviors. In fact guys, chicks often dig a man who has a sensitive side. That said, in my experience, mindless eating is often recognized and more readily confessed to by both genders. Lots of us do it, only we are afraid to acknowledge or talk about it.

An Issue with Many Names

Disordered eating can range in severity and intensity, affecting people differently. It can range from severe binge eating episodes to occasional overeating. Emotional eating, stress-eating, binge eating, compulsive eating, overeating, mindless eating and eating due to food addiction are all considered disordered eating patterns. Binge Eating Disorder and Night Eating Syndrome are two eating disorders that contain disordered eating patterns. Regardless of the severity or intensity of your disordered eating, you can work on your thought processes to achieve a healthier relationship with food. There is a quiz in the Appendix in the back of this book that you can take to help determine if you have a healthy relationship with food.

What Disordered Eating is NOT

Admitting that you struggle with disordered eating is not a copout. People who have food issues do not go around saying they have an addiction to food and use it as an excuse to eat. If anything, they probably hate food. They feel like food is the enemy because they know they cannot stop overindulging. That's how I felt. Many people who suffer from disordered eating often don't taste and enjoy their food. They are caught up in feeling bad about eating and they barely realize they are doing it.

Food addiction is not less serious than other addictions. Not being able to control your food intake leads to excess weight, which is a risk factor for other diseases such as diabetes, heart disease and some cancers. (Barry, Clarke, & Petry, 2009) Also, people with addictive personalities often withdraw into themselves, which can have a negative impact on their quality of life. People with addictions can get lost within themselves and lose relationships along the way. Clearly, food addiction can have both negative physical and mental consequences.

Disordered eating patterns do not develop overnight, thus you cannot "fix" them overnight. Addictive tendencies may be ingrained in you. It may seem impossible to overcome them. Be patient with yourself. You've had an unhealthy relationship with food for a long time and it will take a long time to change. The more you become aware of your habits, the more you will understand why you do what you do. For many things in life, if you learn why you do something, it is easier to learn how to change it.

People with disordered eating patterns often don't recognize they have a problem. It took me a long time to realize that I had issues with food. It took longer to admit that it was a serious problem and to try to get help. Here is the journal entry from when I finally admitted I had a problem controlling myself:

5.26.05

Hi, my name is Julie and I am addicted to food. I have a food addiction. I have a food addiction? Let me get out my Webster's to verify. Addiction – the state of being enslaved to a habit or practice or to something that is psychologically or physically habit-forming, as narcotics, to such an extent that its cessation causes severe trauma. Severe trauma? Hmmm… does it interfere with my life? Absolutely. Ok. I have a food addiction.

So, what the hell do I do now? Took me a whole year to say it out loud, write it down, and say it to someone I know. It still sounds funny. Addiction is a word that sounds very harsh. The phrase "food addiction" makes me cringe. To stick a word like food, something everyone needs every day of his or her life, next to a word like addiction sounds strange. Food addiction? Yes. Air addiction? No. Water addiction? No. Food addiction. Yes.

Emotional eating sounds more pleasant. Compulsive eating sounds less pleasant but not quite as disturbing as food addiction. You cannot get away from food. You need it. You don't need crack, speed, weed, alcohol, cigarettes or other things people usually associate with addictions. People can go their whole lives without these things. However, you need food. I have to learn to control something I need every day.

I've been trying to control my eating my whole life. I have failed. I can go for quite some time without my trigger foods but as soon as something bad happens, it's like I forget everything I know about food and I just shove my face.

I thought Gram was going to die a couple of weeks ago. I spent a week going right up to Scranton after work to see her in ICU. I was exhausted and hungry by the time I left the hospital so I went out to eat every day. I had Chinese, Italian, Wendy's, Cracker Barrel, Smokey Bones, and more Chinese. My spoon, peanut butter, and chocolate chips became my best friend every night before bed. I felt like I lost control.

I bought a book that was published by Psychology Today about food addiction. I asked Chet if he would read it with me. I told him I need his help. That was a big step for me. I told him if I am going to keep it under control, we have to make big changes in our house with food.

Unfortunately, he likes lots of junky food. It is too accessible in our house. If he wants to eat junk, I want him to do it out of our house. He looked like I shot his puppy or something when I asked him. If I were an alcoholic he wouldn't keep alcohol in the house, so why should it be different with junk food? *(footnote)

I hope this new book helps. I hope Chet helps. I need help.

My name is Julie and I am addicted to food.

*Note:

Since I wrote this journal entry I have come to understand that I can have foods around me that I would have considered "off limits" without being especially drawn to them. At one time, I did feel like the food called me. Once I learned I could theoretically eat whatever I wanted, it lost its appeal. Food lost its power over me. I know right now you may not fathom that what I'm saying could possibly be true. I swear it is true. If you practice, one day you will sit right next to your favorite foods and 95% of the time you won't reach for them until you are physically hungry and you'll stop eating them when you are satisfied, not stuffed. You will be able to leave some for later once you are satisfied and not eat them again until you choose. The more you explore your relationship with food, the more you may find your tastes change. You may find what you once considered completely seductive you may not enjoy anymore. If you put in the hard work to rewire your thought processes, your whole attitude towards food and yourself will change.

I wrote in my journal several times a week for quite a while. I felt good about putting all my thoughts on paper. It felt cleansing. I felt better when I shared my journal entries with some of my loved ones. I started to reconnect with people again. It made me realize my disordered eating was more serious than I thought. Food controlled my life and I had no control over it. I do now. With a lot of practice, you can too.

One of the Most Important Concepts to Grasp

Our bodies are smart. Our stomach sends our brain signals to let it know when it is hungry and when it is full. If we learn to listen, we will eat when our body needs fuel and stop when we are satisfied. I know the idea sounds simple, but if you've never done it, it can prove quite difficult. In fact, it may sound impossible. The more you practice, the easier it gets. Eventually your body will use its excess weight as fuel and you will reach a healthy weight for your body.

Chapter 8
Self-Image and Positive Thinking

Many people feel awful about themselves. That's no way to live... I know from experience. You've probably been giving yourself negative messages for many, many years. Once you are engrained in your habits it can be quite difficult to turn them around. I know you are looking for me to tell you there is an easy fix, but I'm sorry there is not. You need to work hard to reverse the negativity you have inside yourself. It is absolutely worth it! Consistency is the key. This chapter gives some ideas of how to start that work. The freedom experienced when you feel good about yourself is indescribable.

When your brain is freed of your negative self-talk, it will have room for more productive, positive things.

The beginning of any journey is always the hardest. You need to get warmed up. Once you get started you will be amazed at how easily the changes come. I think one of the best things you can do for yourself is journal. It helped me bring my thoughts and feelings to the surface. Let go and put all your thoughts down in writing... you don't have to share them with anyone if you don't want to.

Don't be afraid of honesty. You will continue to hurt and stunt your growth if you hold it in.

Observe your thoughts throughout the day.

Most of us go through our days hearing the little voice in our heads, but not really paying attention to what it is saying. It is familiar background noise. I was stunned when I looked back at my journal and realized all the negative things that preoccupied my mind. That "fat, stupid, ugly, lazy, worthless" record constantly played at a low volume. I always portrayed myself as a positive person. I guess I fooled everyone, including myself. We all wear a mask sometimes. It is time to take the mask off and start being real, especially with yourself.

I encourage you to take a little notebook around with you for a day and write down some of the things you are telling yourself. Reviewing it can be quite discouraging. You have probably beat yourself up for years, and it is easy to get upset with the person who was being mean to you… you. Try to let it go. Do not beat yourself up for beating yourself up! You can change the messages you send yourself, but it will take time. Be kind to yourself in this process.

Change your focus.

Odds are you've been talking negatively about yourself for so long that you don't know how to compliment yourself. It is easy to call yourself a worthless, fat slob or something of the like, since you are used to doing it. Pick something you like about yourself and concentrate on that. For example, I refused dessert three times this week because I wasn't physically hungry. Ok, so I did eat dessert twice when I was full. I could dwell on that, or I could choose to highlight my accomplishments for the week. I thought to myself, "I'm happy I am taking steps towards ending my emotional eating tendencies and I know I will only get better at it over time." If I'm concentrating on that thought I don't have room in my brain for, "Boy I'm such an idiot for eating those two desserts this week when I wasn't hungry. I'll never get this right."

The more you focus on the positive, the less room you will have to focus on the negative.

It will seem forced in the beginning. You aren't used to doing it yet. You need to make a conscious effort to say as many positive things to yourself as possible throughout the day. Make inspirational signs and hang them up around your house as reminders. You can also tape little notes to your phone or tablet. Negative thoughts have been repeated in your mind over and over and over and over. You need to counteract with positive, thankful thoughts over and over and over and over to get the message across. The more you do it, the more easily it will happen.

Stop obsessing.

People with an unhealthy relationship with food obsess about it. They focus on if they are being "good" or "bad" depending on what they eat. They obsess about their bodies. **Dieting constantly is a sneaky way of continuing obsessive behavior.** If you are thinking about how many calories, grams of carbs, fiber, fat, saturated fat, protein, or using any method of tracking, **you are obsessing about food and you are not thinking about whatever it is that is truly bothering you.** Food and dieting is a distraction from your real life. You don't end up dealing with your emotions, and you don't end up taking time to be happy about the good things either. You end up missing life experiences while you are obsessing. You probably don't only obsess about the food; you probably obsess about what people are thinking and what you think about yourself.

Again, journaling may bring your behaviors to light. Here is a good example about how obsessive I was about food and what people thought of me:

8.19.04

I went to a friend's bridal shower Saturday. Beforehand all I did was worry about how I was going to look, who met me before and knew I blew up like a blimp, wondering if anyone knew that I shaved my face before I got there, what would they think if I ate exactly what I wanted to, how much

was enough food to eat not to be rude and enough
not to look like a pig, how many desserts could I
try without looking like a pig (her mother-in-law
briefed me on all the goodies they made and bought
– some from one of the best local bakeries, how
could they? Don't they know I can never stop
eating that junk?!), was someone going to ask me
if I tried counting carbs for the millionth time?
Could I take food home with me or would I look
like a pig? How about if I pretended that it was
for Chet and pretended to get only things he
liked? (I did do that.) I set up all these
situations and you know what? Nobody gave a hoot!
Didn't see anyone looking at my plate or grimacing
because I took home cookies. Didn't see anyone
mentally add up how many calories I had eaten. The
only thing that did bother me was that I sat next
to the bride when she was opening her presents. I
was probably in every single freaking picture. I
hope they were close-ups and I wasn't in the
photos. Maybe she cut half of my body out of the
shot. Maybe she only got from the waist up so that
nobody would remember that my thighs spread out
approximately four feet when I sat down. Then
again, maybe nobody cared or noticed.

I noticed that I made comments about how I
was going to eat whatever I wanted. When someone
got diet soda I made sure to say that I wanted
regular because I wanted extra carbs and that
nobody was going to stop me from eating those
candies and cake. I was trying to laugh at myself
so that nobody else could laugh first. All I did
was draw attention to myself if anything.

The whole experience could have been as simple as me getting dressed up for a party and enjoying my company and good food. Instead I wasted time and energy on all that negativity in my brain. I don't do that anymore. You don't have to either. Instead of letting yourself spiral downward with negative thinking, stop yourself and switch your thoughts to the positive. For example, instead of thinking, "I wonder what all these people who I haven't seen in a long time are going to think about how fat I have gotten." Change it to, "I'm happy to get to see people I haven't connected with for a while. It will be nice to catch up on what's been going on in their lives."

Practice gratitude.

For example, every night before bed think of three things that you are thankful for or three things that you are proud that you did during the day. Be grateful for all the positive changes you are making. Thinking about positive things before bed will put you in a good frame of mind for your night's rest. Likewise, beginning your day with the same exercise can help you start off on the right track. You will be surprised at how often you focus on thankful thoughts once you start. We all take so much for granted. It is nice to stop and remind ourselves of all that we have.

Accept compliments.

When you have a low self-esteem it is easy to blow off other people's compliments. Thanking people and not coming back with something negative is important. Them: "You're such a pretty girl." You: "Aw, I'm not that pretty." Or "I need to lose weight." Them: "You are so smart." You: "I'm sure others are smarter." Them: "You are nice to be around." You: "You don't know the real me, I can be a jerk". Sound familiar? Whether it's your family, friends, neighbors, or someone in the grocery store line, you need to thank them for the compliment. The more you don't come back with a negative response, the more likely you will be able to believe what people are telling you.

List your good qualities that have nothing to do with your looks.

Stop and write down every good quality you have and everything positive you can possibly think about yourself. Example: I am smart, funny, giving, helpful, loving, a good singer, etc. You will have this list to refer to whenever you are feeling particularly negative to remind yourself of your positive qualities.

Reconnect with your body, accept and appreciate it.

Many of us spend a large amount of time and energy wishing we looked differently. We pick apart our body, dissecting it in our minds until we are virtually unrecognizable to ourselves. I've heard both men and women point out all the negative things about themselves. It's exhausting to listen to. I used to exhaust myself the same way.

I am beautiful. Some of that has to do with the fact that I am what many people would consider pretty. (It literally took me 20 years to know that.) I have thick, shiny hair, decent skin, hazel eyes that look different depending on what I'm wearing, a great smile and naturally pink lips. However, I believe what mostly makes me attractive is my light... my energy. My love for life and people shines and brings people to me. I want to share my joy with as many people as I can, help others see how beautiful they are and help them marvel in the beauty that surrounds us all. I think that is what attracts people the most, not what I look like.

I could easily tear myself apart too. I have an area that is balding in my crown. I have many, many facial hairs because of the PCOS. I have hanging skin all over my body from losing a massive amount of weight. My thighs have dimples. My arms have the batwing effect. My breasts sag. I have lost a lot of weight, but I am still obese… carrying a lot of excess fat. My heels are cracked. Some of my toenails are funky from losing them to blisters and other sports-related toe injuries. I have wrinkles. My speaking voice is quite nasal. Man… this could be my online dating profile, huh? No? Exactly! Why would I choose to highlight all those things?! I wouldn't do that to attract someone else, so why would I do that to myself? Why would I like myself if all I see is all the least attractive qualities I have?

Now flip to the back of the book and look at me. What I described about myself is all true. Is that what you see when you look at me? I'm going to bet it is not. You probably see my glow, my happiness, the sparkle in my eyes and my beautiful smile. If I were trying to attract a mate, to get someone to like me, I certainly wouldn't sit there and point out all of the negative things about myself. The same goes for when you are trying to get you to like you. Start pointing out all the good things.

The light, the happiness, the positive energy is what makes you more attractive to people than any of your physical qualities. What lights you up? What makes you feel alive? That needs to be your focus.

I know what makes me happy. This does…. writing lights me up. Getting all my thoughts down on paper to communicate to you, to potentially help you change the way you think, feeds my soul. To talk to people, to connect with them and bring them understanding and validation. To share life… to marvel in the wonder that surrounds us. To sit and watch the sun dance on the river before me as it sets, making the sky light up with warm pinks, oranges and purples. To listen to the birds sing their songs in the morning as the soft light starts to wake me up, and the cooler air hits the bare skin of my arms as the rest of my body is nice and toasty under my warm, fluffy, soft sheets and comforter. I get to lie and think about what things I get to enjoy today, another day I get to be on this planet. To get to work out and feel myself getting stronger. To sit across from my man and gaze into his sexy greyish-blue eyes while we enjoy a wonderful meal, a glass of wine, some soft music and candlelight. To see my family and share their love. To get their hugs, see their faces, tell stories, joke around and have lots of laughs. To have girl talk time with friends, to talk about everything or nothing. To read a book and get drawn into it or enjoy my favorite TV show. To sing my feelings until I'm done feeling them. There are many things we get to do that we take for granted every single day. If you take the time to notice, you will be happier. You will start to have that glow of enjoying life. You will feel the energy. You will feel beautiful. Then you will get what you always wanted, to be beautiful.

Did you notice that none of what I described had anything to do with what I look like? What lights me up has nothing to do with my physical being.

But I know it is easy to feel disconnected to your body and the media certainly doesn't help:

6.13.07
        Know what I really hate? I absolutely hate those newscasts that talk about the obesity epidemic and whatever new "treatment" is available and the whole time they are showing footage of all these heavy people walking by with their heads cut off the shot. How exactly is that helping? Can we humiliate these people anymore? How would you feel if it was your butt or gut they had a close up on while talking about how high the death rate is among the obese population? Many heavy people feel a disconnection from their bodies. I'm sure that

showing all these people from the neck down is
drilling that into everyone's head... *you are not a
whole person, you are only your fat.* What kind of
programming is that?! Next time they want to show
fat footage I wish they would do a close up on a
whole person. Better yet, how about they don't
show any "fat" footage? I think we all know what
fat looks like, thank you very much!

Our bodies are the homes for our souls. Stop rolling your
eyes... seriously, our bodies are our homes.... it's where we live
every day. If we don't recognize that our bodies are wonderful and
beautiful, we will be less likely to accept them. If you feel
disconnected from your body, you are less likely to want to take
care of it. **The more you learn to connect with and be present
with your body, the more you can connect with your feelings.
The more you are connected with your feelings, the more you
will find healthy ways of expressing them.** If you can allow
yourself to feel and deal with your feelings, you will stop reaching
for food. Your body is yours and your feelings are yours. You need
to get in touch with both in order to heal. You are the only one who
knows how you feel in your skin. You can try some of the things I
did, but it is up to you to shift your thinking:

6.19.07
          I used to be repulsed by my body. When I was
young I remember grabbing handfuls of my fat rolls
and wishing there were a magic machine that you
could use to suck the fat off. Maybe the machine
would pull it off like taffy. Hmmmm... the thoughts
of youth... and just last night. Just kidding. Not
really.

I have finally accepted my body. Accepting my body doesn't mean getting complacent with the fact it will always look the same or I will always be the same weight… but why not accept it for what it is right now since it's not like it will change at lightning speed? It is not like there is a machine that can pull the fat off like taffy, so you need to accept where you are and be comfortable with who you are in your skin, while feeling good about the fact that you are taking steps to have the best body you can have. Besides, *feeling good about yourself looks beautiful no matter what your size.* I feel good. I look good.

[My family may want to skip this paragraph ☺] I had a hard time getting intimate with my husband when we first started dating. I often wondered why my fat stomach, my dimply butt and thighs, or my wiggly arms didn't repulse him. I would cringe when he would touch those parts and try to shoo him to a less repulsive body part. I gained a lot of weight the first four years we were together, almost 150 pounds, and it only got worse over time. I stopped wanting to be naked in front of him. I didn't want the lights on if I was naked. Truth is I was lucky enough to have a husband who loved me no matter what my weight was… all of this negativity came solely from me. Over time I realized I had to change how I felt about my body for me… it had nothing to do with Chet or anyone else.

I started to focus on feeling good in my skin. I started wearing skirts and realized my legs didn't look that bad. I felt very feminine. I started wearing tank tops even though my stretch marks showed on my shoulders. Those stupid stretch marks made me feel hideous for years. I got over it. I stopped wearing a T-shirt in the pool to cover myself up- something I had done my entire life. When I was in the shower I would look at my body as I washed. I would be thankful for all the muscle I built up under those fat rolls and I learned to appreciate how strong I was physically – after all, I worked out consistently for years.

I felt better when I started going for monthly massages. I started going for massages because I passed out a couple years ago, smashed my face on the floor, and wrecked my neck. I was getting severe knots in my back that would cause me to get migraines all the time and my chiropractor recommended massage to get the kinks out. It worked wonders... but the massages did something more than get rid of my migraines. I started getting more parts of my body massaged over time and I realized I'd cringe or have negative body image thoughts throughout the hour. Over time I became more and more comfortable in my skin. I was more relaxed than I had ever been. Being that relaxed *while* someone touched my body helped me associate being comfortable while being touched. There was a time I'd cringe getting a hug from someone because they touched my back fat rolls. I finally realized that people aren't hugging my fat, they are hugging me! I am not my fat! It's been an amazing internal transformation.

Also, I started meditating after I exercise. I do deep breathing while mentally doing a body scan (focusing on different parts, starting with my toes and going up to my head) while being proud of all the work I've done to get my body as strong as it is... it's made a big difference.

Look in the mirror and identify traits about yourself that you like.

Sometimes it is easier to come up with intangible things we like about ourselves. It is important to look at your physical traits and focus on what you like about yourself as well. Maybe you like your hair or your lips. Maybe you think your eyes are beautiful or that you have a pretty smile. Focus on positive things and be thankful for them and ignore the negative.

[Ok Julia, you had me until this one. Really? You expect ME to sit here and look at myself and find something I like? You know I haven't liked anything about myself in a very long time, if ever, now that I think about it. Why on earth would you expect me to be able to do this?!] You didn't know I could read your mind, did you? Well, I know this may be the hardest thing for you to do, but please, for your own good, give it the best shot you can. Practice this every day until you no longer get disgusted by looking in the mirror.

Meditate/Use Positive Mantras

The first time I thought about meditating I thought about someone sitting in an empty room with their legs crossed in a way I certainly couldn't cross them, chanting to themselves. Meditation can be whatever you make it. It can be five minutes of closing your eyes and being mindful of your breath, or it can be a half hour of repeating positive messages to yourself. When I have excessive negative thoughts floating through my brain, I take it as a sign that I need to pause. I breathe deeply and repeat to myself "in with the good" as I inhale through my nose and "out with the bad" as I exhale through my mouth. Experiment with different ways of breathing to see what works best for you. There are videos on the internet that can teach you different breathing and meditation techniques. A yoga studio in your area can also help. Check around to see if anyone holds meditation classes.

Many people are shallow breathers. A deep breath should fill your lower lungs (your belly will rise) and your upper lungs (your chest will rise). If you are busy repeating those simple words (inhale - "in with the good", exhale - "out with the bad"; inhale - "I am", exhale - "just this") as you breathe deeply your brain can't think about the negative. You will feel refreshed. You will get better at it over time. Each time your mind wanders, bring it back to your breath and positive phrases.

Examples of positive mantras:
- My weight does not determine my mood.
- The more I do, the more I can do.
- Moving is better than not moving.
- "CAN'T" is not in my vocabulary.
- I am feeling healthier every day.
- Nothing feels better than strong.
- I am so thankful for all that I have in my life... my friends, family, job, food, shelter, car, clothing, etc.

If you intentionally repeat these mantras you will burn good messages into your brain. Come up with positive mantras that have special meaning to you. You can start with "I am _____ " and fill in the blank with anything positive; smart, sexy, funny, giving, loving, a good friend, a nurturing mother, a supportive wife, etc. Make a little sign to hang in places you frequent (mirror in the bathroom, by your PC or TV, or on your nightstand). Every time you pass the sign you can repeat the mantra several times to help remind you to stay positive. Yes, I realize it may seem weird to people that come to your home, but remember, LOTS of people fight negative thoughts. Your positive messages may inspire others in your life to start being nice to themselves as well!

Realize that you shouldn't care about what other people think about you.

Something important I learned is that other people are too worried about what you think about them to worry about you. For example, people are paranoid about going to the gym. They often stop themselves from going because they feel people are watching and criticizing. Most of the time people focus on their own workouts or their own paranoia. They probably are not paying attention to you. We all deserve to use a gym. The purpose is to get into better physical shape, which people of all sizes and fitness levels need. The grocery store was also a tough place for me. I would feel like people were looking in my shopping cart, judging my purchases. The people in the grocery store do not know you. Why should their opinion of your food bother you? And again, they are probably not paying attention to you anyway.

Stop waiting until you are "skinny" to do things you've always wanted to do.

You know what I mean… you think you need to lose weight before you can dance, sing, hike, etc. Think about what you would like to do and do it now. Your weight will only hold you back if you let it… start living right now! Can you think of things you've been holding off on doing until you are thinner? Go to the beach? Wear a swimsuit? Write down things you've been holding back from doing. Make it one of your goals to do whatever that thing is at your current weight if it is physically possible, and it's not your mind holding you back.

Get clothes you feel attractive in.

Clothes shopping sucks, no matter what your size. There are many different body types out there and unfortunately the fit model your designer used probably isn't your type. Put the time in to try on outfits until you find that one that you feel amazing in. You know that feeling you get when you like how you look in your clothes… you stand taller, you smile a little brighter. You are worth having clothes that make you feel that good. If you do your best, but still can't find anything you like, you can have clothes tailored. I know it sounds expensive. However, if you have pants that would make your butt look awesome but they are four inches too long, wouldn't it be worth the eight dollars to shorten them? You don't need to go out and buy a whole new wardrobe, but you can make yourself feel better by getting a couple outfits you feel great in. After feeling bad about yourself for so long you deserve it!

Take some "me" time.

Shut off your phone. Don't check your email. Relax. Take a bubble bath, light candles, read, meditate, go for a leisurely walk, enjoy fresh air, sing, dance, soak your feet, get a massage, or just sit. I don't care what you do, but you should make time for yourself every single day. I know that can be hard, especially for those that have a nurturing personality, but if you don't recharge yourself you won't be any good for anyone else. It is hard to feel good about yourself if you feel overextended all the time. Start with a short amount of time if this one seems like it will be difficult. Don't you have at least 15-20 minutes you can dedicate to yourself? Nobody will give you the time… you have to take it.

Don't compare yourself to others.

We are all running our own races. We need to set our own goals and do our own personal best. Everyone is dealt a different set of cards. It is not fair to compare yourself to other people since everyone's situation isn't the same. Looks can be deceiving... you may wish your life were like someone else's, but you never know what it's like to walk in their shoes. Be proud of the effort you are putting forth and strive to make **you** better. You will win *your* race with that attitude.

Slow Down.

We spend our time living our life in high gear. We barely notice what we are doing, whether it's eating, exercising, or anything else. **How you perceive your time often has a bigger impact on your outlook.** For example, you know you only have 15 min at work for a break to eat your snack. Do you rush through it? How can you enjoy it or feel satisfied if you barely paid attention to what you were doing? If you took your time chewing and enjoying your food it probably wouldn't take 15 minutes to eat it anyway.

```
4.09.06
        When I am eating emotionally I do it very
fast. I shove my face until there is no food left.
I don't taste it. I don't really enjoy it. That
same kind of rushing through the task applies to
so many other things I do.
        When I come home from work there are so many
things I want to do: exercise, cook, eat dinner,
shower, write, email, watch my favorite shows,
etc. I feel like there is not enough time to do
everything I want. All that means is that when I
pick the first thing, say exercise, I get right to
it - get dressed as fast as I can, get out the
door as fast as I can, walk as fast as I can,
stretch as fast as I can, lift as fast as I can,
stretch again, etc. Then I heat up the food as
```

fast as I can, eat as fast as I can, clean the table off and make my lunch as fast as I can, etc. Then I might sit down to write in my journal and type as fast as I can. Everything is "as fast as I can". It makes me tired. I don't end up enjoying anything I do since I am worried about what I need to do next, and next, and next...(close your eyes, take a deep breath and...sigh).

Once I start doing something I feel like I better do a lot of it since it might be a while until I have time to do it again. If I am eating, I eat a lot. If I am drinking, I drink a lot. If I am exercising, I exercise a lot. If I am writing, I write a lot. If I am reading, I read a lot. For example, I read a book recently that my sister loaned me two years ago. I never got to read it since I haven't been doing any "fun" reading. Everything I read is about PCOS, food, or exercise. Once I started reading I sat there for most of the day since I figured I better read the whole thing in one sitting. It took me two freaking years to pick up the damn book but I *had to* spend a whole day reading it in case I didn't get to pick it up again anytime soon. I didn't enjoy the latter half of the book. I kept turning the page, reading too fast, and telling myself that if I go a little faster I will have the whole thing done in no time. Why couldn't I have read for a half hour every night for a week instead and enjoyed it?

So, last week I posted signs that said "SLOW DOWN". I ate slower and enjoyed the taste of my food. I didn't end up eating as much. I read slower and enjoyed reading. I exercised slower, taught my husband about good form, and enjoyed exercising. I enjoyed the fresh air and sunshine while we were walking. I enjoyed how my body felt after we walked and stretched. I thought about each muscle group as I stretched and appreciated all that I have done so far to get in shape. When we lifted I enjoyed challenging myself with higher weights, or reps, or by going slower. I appreciated what I was doing for myself. I enjoyed everything. And guess what? It didn't take me any longer to do any of it! It was my perception that changed; I felt dramatically different.

Reward Yourself.

A little positive reinforcement never hurts. Problem is, many of us reward ourselves with food. Try to think of non-food rewards. Believe me, I know that can be asking a lot. For example, give yourself some extended "me" time. Take a whole afternoon for yourself! It is free, but many of us don't do it. You could get yourself a movie, a book, a CD, a face mask, a new lotion, etc. The bigger your goals, the bigger your rewards should be… like if you exercised 5 days a week for 8 weeks, you promise to go out and buy new sneakers, workout clothes or maybe get a massage.

Spread the positive energy.

It may be one of the most important things you do. If the people around you feel good about themselves, they will emit positive energy too and everyone benefits. Whenever an opportunity arises give others compliments and signs of affection…. when appropriate of course. (That reminded me of my Mom telling me about my first kiss. I believe I was two and apparently decided this little boy next to us in a restaurant looked like he could go for a kiss. Guess I've never been shy!) Who doesn't like a big smile or a good hug? Isn't it the case that when you are out in public and flash someone those pearly whites, you often get them to smile in return?

Life can be hard enough without someone constantly pulling you down. If key players in your life tend to be negative, try explaining to them how you are trying to change your thought processes and see if they would like to work on it as well. You can become cheerleaders for each other.

Exercise.

Exercise raises the feel-good chemicals in your body and helps lower stress. Feeling stronger makes it easier to develop a positive body image. You can connect to and like/enjoy a body that you have been putting the hard work into. I feel passionate about exercise and all its benefits. Please review the Chapter 15: Get Moving! And get off the couch! The more you move, the more you can move... the better you will feel!

Forgive.

Once you realize your behaviors are self-destructive, it is easy to continue beating yourself up and abusing yourself. It might not make sense unless you've done it, but once you realize the pain you've been causing yourself, you may get angry, depressed, frustrated, etc. The only way, until now, that you've dealt with those types of feelings is to eat. You may eat more once you identify the problem. You may get mad at yourself if you feel you've encouraged this behavior in others. You may get upset with those from whom you feel you learned your behavior. You may not want to be around people with whom you have overeaten. You may get mad at our society or the state of the world today for setting us up for addiction. Accept that you didn't have the tools up until recently to behave any differently than you've been behaving. You are a work in progress.

Forgive: there is no room for negativity when you are trying to heal.

Never give up on yourself!

I know you are a strong person. If you have been struggling with negative thoughts and your weight your whole life, you had to be strong. You have been mistreating yourself for a long time. You've been struggling with the negative thoughts in your head. Maybe it's hard to get through the day. You've had to fight to get off the couch, to go up a flight of stairs, to fit into seats, to get your chores done or keep up with your personal hygiene. Like me, you have been fighting for a long time.

You can choose a different fight. Fight to change your thought processes. Fight to learn healthy coping mechanisms. Fight to become more active and fit. You can do this. You deserve to live a better life.

Chapter 9
Rewiring Your Thinking

This chapter focuses on the "why"," how" and "when" of your eating habits and learning new, healthier behaviors. I wish I could tell people that it would be a "quick fix". I wish I could say "sure you feel like crap about yourself today, but by next week you'll be a new person". Nope... isn't going to happen that way. Odds are you've had a dysfunctional relationship with food for years and it may take quite a while to repair it. However, that doesn't mean you won't notice and appreciate all the small, positive changes along the way.

For me, the hardest part about my progress over the last few years is that it cannot be measured; it's been about quality not quantity. You could look at a picture of me from two, three, or four years ago and you would not see all the changes I've made internally. Yes, at the time I wrote this chapter I had already lost 90 pounds. However, I haven't lost much in the last few years, even though the most change in my thinking occurred during this time. ***Your journey is not about losing weight, it is about learning about you and loving yourself.*** Ultimately, you will change your behaviors and thought processes; weight loss should occur over time, even though it is not the primary focus. I know that sounds ridiculous because it has probably been your focus for years. Please remind yourself where that type of thinking got you so far. It's time to try something new.

Everyone is different and may go through the process in a different order. The important thing to ask yourself is if you are ready to follow through with each step. If you act prematurely, you may fall back into your old habits, feeling defeat. If you wait until you are ready, you will be more likely to make the changes last forever.

Only you can determine which steps are appropriate for you at any given time. Don't forget you can do more than you think you can. Don't avoid trying something because it is new and scary.

I hope you find comfort in knowing that I understand what you go through every day. Make the commitment to yourself to keep moving forward no matter how frustrated you get. You are the only one who can change you. The first step can be admitting that what you've tried in the past has not worked for you.

Acknowledge that diets do not work and what you will be doing is not a diet.

There is a reason people keep coming up with new diets all the time – it's because the market is there. If diets truly did work, there would be no reason for a new diet craze. I'm not saying people don't lose weight on diets, but we all know what happens when you go off them. All too often we end up gaining more than we lost because we didn't learn how to change our negative behaviors. Let me say it again... *you will NEVER have to "diet" again if you work on your relationship with food*. You won't count calories, carbs, protein, fiber, exchanges, etc. ever again because it won't be necessary. You can learn how to eat when you are physically hungry and stop when you are satisfied. You will teach yourself healthy ways to cope with your emotions instead of using food to mask your feelings.

List all of the different diets you have tried that have failed you and all the pounds you have gained, lost, and regained. Acknowledge the frustration of your yo-yo dieting. Decide for yourself if it's worth continuing that pattern, or if you want to make positive, internal changes that will transform your life forever. You can decide to stop dieting today and never diet again. As scary as that sounds, once you make that decision you will start to feel a new sense of freedom.

Realize that it will take time, hard work, and commitment.

When you can finally see your disordered eating patterns and degrading internal dialog, it can be quite overwhelming. I know you can change because I have. I know you are a strong person; you had to be. Only a strong person can handle getting beat up every day, whether it was by others, your internal dialog, or both. You can stop beating yourself up. You can use that strength for change.

What if I told you that five years from now your life could be completely different? You will not beat yourself up. You will be full of positive self-talk. You will be healthier. Your life will not be dictated by food. You will not hide your eating. You will know how to handle emotionally charged situations without turning to food. You will be stronger. You will reap more benefits from your changes in thinking than you can imagine. Wouldn't it be worth whatever you had to do to be free? Wouldn't it be worth the promise and commitment? **Promise yourself you are going to keep working on it for as long as it takes. Consistency is key.**

Sometimes you may get frustrated, but that is only normal. Changing your whole way of thinking about food and your self-image isn't easy. Stop burying your feelings. Bring them to the surface:

`6.26.06`

> I have averaged at least 45 hours a week since January at work. I have tried to keep exercising three times a week, even if it is only to walk for 20 or 30 minutes. I have been working on my food addiction, which takes a ton of energy. Bringing such a big problem to the surface is *exhausting*. It is ALWAYS on my mind. EVERY TIME I think I am hungry I have to ask myself if it is physical hunger or something else. While I am

doing all of this, I am still trying to spend time with my family, friends, and Chet AND write my book! I have been trying to write a little every day. All of this together is too much sometimes. I put an extreme amount of pressure on myself. It is hard to write a book about something you are still trying to figure out for yourself. I need to give myself credit. I need to chill. I can do this.

Realize that everyone is unique and will progress at different rates.

I know you are wondering how long it will take to heal from your food addiction. I can't give you an answer. Everyone's journey is different. The important thing to remember is that you are making changes that are going to make you a healthier person for THE REST OF YOUR LIFE. If you knew it would take you several years to heal from emotional eating, but after that time you would maintain your healthy relationship with food for the next twenty, thirty, forty, or fifty years, wouldn't it be worth the wait? Be patient with yourself. **Don't let the scale determine how you feel**.

Every time I weighed myself, the result was the same... I'd eat! If I gained a pound, I'd eat since "What's the point?!... I screwed up already anyway". If I lost a pound, I'd eat since "I get to celebrate my success... I deserve a treat". Sound familiar? Your focus right now is not your weight, it is on building a better relationship with food and yourself.

I stopped weighing myself and I feel great. I don't let that number get in my head and cause a change in my mood. I understand I am overweight but I have been working hard for years. A number on a scale cannot erase that progress. I am stronger and more physically and emotionally fit. **I use my increasing fitness and how I feel as a meter of my success.** When people start to eat more nutritious foods and exercise, they expect a dramatic change in the scale. That behavior sets you up for failure since weight loss is often slow. If you think you should be losing weight faster it can discourage you. Remember, muscle is denser than fat; if you have been exercising and you stayed the same weight, you may have shifted the proportion of muscle and fat while losing inches. The scale may disagree with how good you feel. Forget about the scale!

It was hard for me when I first started:

04.15.06

I went to my doctor the other day for my weekly weigh in. I told her I didn't want to weigh anymore because of all I learned and recognized about myself this past couple weeks. She wanted to weigh me to record it in my file but she wouldn't tell me. This is the first time in my life I don't have an exact number to go by. I haven't been weighed in almost two weeks. How am I supposed to know how I feel if I don't have that number? How am I supposed to gauge my successes or failures without that number? We talked for several minutes after I jumped off the scale and all I could think in the back of my mind was 'I wonder what I weighed' and 'I probably gained a bunch of weight, that is why she is concerned'.

Not weighing myself was extremely difficult in the beginning:

4.21.06

It has been a week since I told my doctor I wasn't going to weigh myself. I have felt like such a fat pig. Not knowing the number has made me incredibly nervous. Every day I wake up and look in the mirror to see how fat my face is, as if overnight I could have gained twenty pounds. Do I have cheekbones? How big is my double chin? This shirt makes my middle stomach fat roll stick out…etc, etc…every day this week, every hour, all day long.

(Note: if you were told by your physician that you must weigh yourself daily because of problems with fluid retention, please continue. Try your best not to associate a feeling with that number.)

Get rid of the good food/ bad food idea.

I touched on this in an earlier chapter, but it is an important concept. All food is primarily made of carbon, oxygen, hydrogen and some nitrogen atoms. Food is our source of energy. When our body is breaking it down, it doesn't care where the atoms come from. However, the main difference is that some foods have more fiber, vitamins and minerals. Those are the foods us dietitians call nutritionally dense foods. If you listen to your body, you'll find it feels better when you eat nutritionally dense foods, such as fruits and veggies.

The list of what foods are "bad" changes, often depending on the popular diet at the time. Some of those foods may not be made of the best building blocks for your body, but you can eat them in moderation. If you eat slowly and savor each bite, you will not be driven to overindulge, regardless of what food you are eating. Once you give yourself permission to eat, you may find those forbidden foods aren't as good you thought.

8.22.2004

At a grocery store up by Gram's house as soon as you walk in there are Welch cookies to the right. I've been avoiding buying them for at least a year. How goofy is that? I probably ended up at

that store a couple times a month for the last
year. That's at least twenty-four times I wanted
those stupid cookies and I refused to buy them
because they were nothing but carbs and lard.
That's why they taste so good! It was freeing to
buy them and eat them and not feel guilty. I don't
even know how to describe it. I only ate two. In
the past, I may have had 6 or more and then felt
horrible about it. I was more than satisfied with
those two cookies. Gram was thrilled I got them
too, as they are one of her favorites.

I went grocery shopping on my way home from
Gram's and I bought things I've been wanting for
quite some time. That's all I bought — forbidden
foods! First I picked up orange creamsicle soda.
I've wanted that soda for years and didn't let
myself purchase any. [Side note — I threw one
bottle out in the Summer of 2007 since I still had
one. Strange how I thought about it for a long
time and now I haven't had one in 3 years!] Then I
got more mac and cheese and I put butter in it and
everything! I was hungry when I ate it — my
stomach was growling, that's how I know; it's a
new feeling. I stopped when I was almost full. I'm
saving room for later for the donuts I bought.
This brand of donuts has looked good and so did
the chocolate cake. I haven't gotten that cake in
a long time even though it is Chet's favorite,
since I would usually end up taking a fork to it.
Anyhow, all those treats made their way into my
basket and I only heard my voices a little bit.
Mostly they were telling me 'if anybody had a
problem with what was in my basket they could kiss
my… whoa, be nice Jule', etc. Amazingly enough, I
brought all that food home and I ended up not

eating it all in one sitting. I didn't even open it all. I don't know what I am so afraid of. Do I think that the food will fly out of their wrappers and down my throat like it's something I have no control over? Yes.

You may eat food you thought you shouldn't eat for a while, and then you will get over it:

8.28.04

All those foods I mentioned in my last entry looked so good when I thought I couldn't have them. Now that they are in my house, I could care less. It's amazing! When I gave myself permission to eat this junk, I found myself wanting watermelon, cheese, peaches, soup - good foods. Not to say that I don't want junk, but if I do, I don't shovel in the whole box, bag, or package. I don't have to because I am allowed to have some later, tomorrow, next week, or whenever!

People always want what they can't have. Once they get it, they have a smorgasbord and don't find themselves wanting it anymore. Like if you saw this man or women that looked good to you and you spend all your time fantasizing about them. You picture yourself unwrapping them and doing things you might not necessarily say out loud. You chase and chase, if you finally get them, you do what you wanted, it's over before you know it and then you look at them and you don't want them anymore. Sometimes you wish you never did it in the first place and then you feel dirty and swear it won't happen again. It is exactly the same with food. The packages look so colorful and

shiny. You fantasize about unwrapping them. You do
the nasty deed, eat and eat, and then it's over
and you don't want it anymore. You wish you never
did it in the first place and you feel dirty. You
swear you will never do it again. Sometimes it is
about the chase for the forbidden.

Part of the solution is to give yourself permission to eat all
foods. You think I'm crazy, right? I thought that suggestion was
crazy too until I tried it. The key is to eat when you are physically
hungry and stop when you are almost full. It sounds simple, but for
those of us with emotional eating tendencies, it can prove to be
quite a challenge.

**Take the quiz found in the appendix and put your answers in
writing.**

Answer each question honestly, expanding on your answers.
For example, #12 reads, "Do you eat in secret?" For me, for a long
time, the answer was yes. I ate the most when my friends weren't
around or my husband was at work. I ate in the car. I ate late at
night when everyone else slept. I could probably come up with more
examples, but you get the idea. Your answers may surprise you
once you think about it. However, recognizing your behavior is the
start of your journey. Putting your answers down on paper will help
make them more real for you. It's easier to ignore your thoughts if
they are bouncing around in your mind, instead of in black and
white before your eyes.

Acknowledge that you have a dysfunctional relationship with food.

By now you may be kicking around the idea that you struggle with food issues. However, you need to *own* the fact that you have a serious problem. Journaling helps to show you what, when, how, with whom, and your feelings while you eat. Originally, I started my journal to record how PCOS affected my life. After a year I looked back to see what I wrote about. I couldn't believe that all I wrote about was food and how it made me feel! Every day it was the same story. I ate too much... I felt bad about myself... I ate more... I went to the store to buy more... I felt like everyone judged me... I bought more food... I ate more... I felt worse. The cycle went on and on and on and on. I felt like a broken record. I had written a hundred pages only about food!

Until I looked at it in black and white, I would have never thought I had a real problem with food. I thought it was normal behavior for someone who had to lose weight. I thought I was "watching what I ate". I was watching it... I was watching it go right into my mouth! I felt so out of control.

Sometimes if you don't want to admit how you feel out loud you may want to write it down. You don't have to show anyone. I've written my thoughts on paper to get them out of my system. If I don't want anyone else seeing them or I have felt guilty about writing them, I've torn them up and thrown them out. It may take journaling for a while to realize what a serious impact your relationship with food has on your life. It was freeing to admit that I had a problem and I wanted help to change it. This realization finally got me pointed in the right direction. I could finally move forward. It will do the same for you.

What does physical hunger feel like to you?

Take time to figure that out. Throughout the day think about the feeling you have right before you are about to eat. Can you tell if it is physical hunger or if you are eating for other reasons? Describe physical hunger. How is it different from the other times you would like to eat?

Use all your senses as you eat.

When I lead people through an exercise in mindful eating I like to use a clementine. First, use your eyes to appreciate how it looks… the beauty of the different shades of orange, the neat little pores that let the gases flow in and out of the fruit. Appreciate all the work that went into bringing this clementine to your table. As you peel it, notice the spray of the juices as you pick up the wonderful citrus fragrance. Note the pattern the white forms against the orange. When you taste a section, feel the juice squirt into your mouth and taste the wonderful sweetness. As you chew, note how the taste changes. Does it become more bitter? Do you like that? I often like to close my eyes to make sure I am using my full sense of taste. Obviously, this cannot happen all the time, but having your eyes closed eliminates the distraction of your surroundings. We are often searching for that next bite, instead of paying attention to what is happening in our mouths. Use your awareness to see if you enjoy the aftertaste. If you do, you don't have to rush into the next bite or wash it down with your drink. Pause for a moment, then take your next bite. If you eat this slowly, with this much attention, you can tap into the feeling of satisfaction. It is too difficult to tell if you are full if you mindlessly eat, so you certainly can't tell if you are satisfied. How different is an experience like I've described compared to how you normally eat?

The Hunger Scale

We all have times when we eat until we are overstuffed. Think about how you've often felt after Thanksgiving dinner or another holiday meal. If that is the fullest you have felt, you can call that a 10… which translates to feeling sick to your stomach. On the other extreme, have you found yourself so busy that you honestly forgot to eat during the day? That feeling when your stomach is rumbling like crazy and you are nauseous we can call a 1. A 5 would be neutral… you are neither hungry nor full. If you were to eat a snack it wouldn't make you overstuffed, but if you skipped a snack you probably wouldn't notice for a while. It is best to avoid either extreme, but also make sure you don't graze all day and keep yourself in that middle range. When I practiced using the hunger scale, I was surprised to notice how little food it took for me to be satisfied.

Hunger Scale:

10 - I ate so much I'm sick!

9 - If I eat another bite I might be sick.

8 - Uncomfortably full

7- Slightly uncomfortable

6- Perfectly satisfied

5- Neutral – not feeling hungry or full

4- Slightly hungry

3- Tummy is rumbling, it's time to eat!

2- Very hungry – I know I should have eaten a while ago

1- So hungry I'm sick to my stomach!

Record daily food log entries to start being mindful of your eating.

List the time you ate, the approximate quantity, and the people you were with while you ate. Rank your hunger before and after you ate and the feelings you had before and after you ate. When you look back on your entries *do not judge yourself or beat yourself up*! You may be shocked by what you see, but recognizing your behavior is one of the first steps to changing it. You will begin to see your eating patterns and many areas in which you can change to better your health. It may seem quite overwhelming, but don't panic! You'll successfully identify opportunities for improvement. You will then take one step at a time to make those improvements. The next page has a sample food log for you to model yours after.

Example of a Daily Food Log:

Date: _____

Time	Food	Hunger Before	Hunger After	Location/ Company	Feelings Before	Feelings After
9 AM	Egg & cheese on a bagel, 2 donuts, coffee	2	10, over-stuffed	Coffee shop / husband	Happy, Beautiful morning	Sad, ate too much again
11 AM	Small Yogurt	5	8	Couch/ nobody	Antsy	Antsy, wasn't hungry
1 PM	One hot dog, handful of fries, iced T	2	6	Hot dog stand/ family	Peaceful	Peaceful, ate until satisfied
3 PM	Handful of nuts	4	6	Computer/ nobody	Tired	Tired, need a nap
6 PM	12 shrimp, ½ baked sweet potato, salad, broc and cauliflower, iced T	2	7	Kitchen Table/ brother	Amped, worked all day	Satisfied, nice ending to a busy day
11 PM	½ c ice cream	4	5	Couch/ nobody	Tired	Tired, time for bed

I suggest doing the food log until you identify areas you can improve upon: keeping your hunger levels away from the extremes, breaking the connection between certain people or places and food, etc. There is a lot of valuable information in the log. However, it is not something you should obsess over since any obsession can replace your addiction, thus not solving the problem at all.

As shown in this sample food log, I stuffed myself in the morning, ate a few times when I wasn't hungry, ate when I wasn't hungry only when I was by myself, felt bad after eating more than my fill, etc. You have to identify your pattern of behavior first before you can find alternate solutions. Now I come up with healthier ways to feel better besides reaching for food, like going to sit outside for a while to get fresh air and sunshine, taking a walk, or taking a small nap to refresh myself. However, that first step is identifying the behavior you'd like to change. You will learn ways to honor other reasons you eat besides physical hunger, like fatigue or boredom. Later steps will help you find ways to cope with feelings in a healthy way as well.

Learn about your *emotional eating triggers* and how to deal with your emotions/emotionally charged situations in a healthy way.

By journaling or talking with someone, a friend or a professional, you will figure out your emotional eating triggers. People eat because they are depressed, lonely, angry, frustrated, worried, etc. The more you pay attention to your feelings, the more you will be able to express them. Once you identify and express your feelings, you will find ways to deal with your emotions besides eating to numb them.

This next exercise is something that helped me a lot. For a while I wrote down my answers. I carried a little notebook around with me. Then it became automatic.

The Hungry Form:
I am hungry. Am I hungry?

_____

If not, what do I need or want to do about it?

_____

_____

What am I going to do?

_____

Answer these questions honestly. Think about the answers and give yourself time. The answer to the last question may continue to be to eat something when you are not physically hungry for a while. Give yourself a break. You will learn to do healthier things to deal with your emotions in time.

Come up with a list of coping mechanisms you know work for you. Do you like to talk, walk, dance, sing, paint, draw, hit a punching bag, hike, meditate, take a bubble bath, paint your nails, organize your house, journal, email someone you care about, listen to music, enjoy the outdoors, read, play video games, garden, etc.? Sometimes realizing how you feel and why you feel that way is enough. It is ok just to feel.

I used this form often in the beginning and it tapered off over time. I still use it in my head when I am feeling hungry but I am not sure about my hunger's origins. Here is an example of when I first used this exercise:

04.19.06

I have a hard time deciding when I am physically hungry. I think that I associate guilt with hunger so I let my mind block when I am physically hungry. I think it is also a control issue; I force myself to not feel hungry when I am

physically hungry, so later when I am emotionally
hungry I can shove my face.

I made a form about hunger. It says: I am
hungry. Am I hungry? Why? What do I need or want
to do about it? What am I going to do? I have it
on my computer table and dining room table so it
can help me think before I eat. I sit there and
write the answers to slow myself down sometimes.
If I am emotionally eating, it will help me
realize I have a choice. I might end up eating; I
might not. However, I will be clear on what I am
doing and it will help me get in touch with my
true feelings. If I am physically hungry, it will
help me realize I can take my time, figure out
what I want, and take the time to make it. The
hardest part for me is when I am physically hungry
but upset about something at the same time. I need
to learn to separate the two types of hunger,
allow myself the food I want to satisfy the
physical hunger, decide what I can do to satisfy
the emotional hunger, while not mistaking
physically feeling full with emotionally taking
care of myself.

Even the question of "what do I want to
eat?" is hard for me to answer. I think it goes
back to feeling guilty about the food; I don't
want to choose things I know are "bad". That is
probably why answering the question "what do I
want?" has been very difficult. If I don't allow
myself to choose food I want to eat, how can I
allow myself to choose what school I want to go
to, what career I'd like to have, or anything else
for that matter?

The hunger form worked last night. Here is an
example: I am hungry. Am I hungry? No. What am I?

Sad/mad. **Why?** Because my knees and feet hurt and I would like to do more walking. My pain is my own fault because I let myself get so big. I am angry with myself. **What do I need or want to do about it?** Have Chet rub my knees, soak my feet, and get new sneakers.

Two minutes later I saw chocolates on the table from Easter. I am hungry. Am I hungry? No, I just went over this. **What am I?** Besides sad/mad I'm thirsty. **What can I do about it?** Have some water.

Learn about your *environmental triggers* and practice changing your behavior.

From my food journal entries, I noticed I always eat when I am on the couch, especially watching TV, and when I am with certain people or at certain places. For example, every time I walked into my Gram's house I thought it was time to eat, regardless of whether or not I was hungry. I always walked right over to the fridge. I think it is because when I was in college I went over to her house for lunch quite often, so when I visited it was time for me to eat. I needed to assess my hunger as soon as I arrived, because if I didn't think about it, I could lose control rather quickly.

It is best to eat at a kitchen or dining room table without distraction – no reading, watching TV, surfing on the internet, checking your phone, etc. It will help bring your attention to your eating. You will enjoy your food more. Again, I often chew with my eyes closed. It is harder to get distracted if you are not looking at other things.

When you review your food log entries, notice if there are any patterns related to where or with whom you eat. Do you eat only until a level of 7 on your fullness scale when you are by yourself and consistently eat until you are a 10 with certain people or in certain places? Do you mindlessly eat while in your car, surfing the internet, watching TV or reading? When you strengthen your awareness, you can work on your behavior during these situations. It will get easier over time to not eat in your car or in front of the TV. You will eventually learn not to associate people or places with food. Eating will stop being something to do to fill the gaps.

Here's when I realized I *always* eat before bed:
8.19.04

My family has always eaten at night, *always*. I remember Thursday nights at eight when the Cosby show was on we would have huge bowls of ice cream. At the time I didn't know they were huge; now that I learned about portion size I know that they were at least three to four servings. That was the pattern every day during the week. Some TV show and some kind of food and then bed. I still do it. I think I like the full feeling. It helps me sleep. I especially like having warm food at night. It is like a warm hug. Like Thanksgiving dinner, you get yourself all stuffed and then you can take a nap, all cozy and warm. I don't want to eat at night anymore, but I can't stop myself yet. I ate a piece of Danish and mac and cheese last night even though I knew I was not hungry. It tasted good. At least I tasted it this time.

Honestly, it took quite a while for me not to eat before bed when I wasn't physically hungry. Instead I've tried hot tea with my nightly TV show. It does get easier the more you practice it... I promise. It is our own choice whether to eat or not to eat when we are not hungry. You will learn that if you eat when you are not hungry you usually end up not feeling well. The more you practice, you will learn not to eat when you are not physically hungry to avoid being sick to your stomach or having heartburn.

Start paying close attention to your hunger.

Determine if you eat because of physical hunger or emotional hunger. Is your stomach growling? Does your tummy feel hallow? If so, you are probably physically hungry. Are you sad about a relationship or angry about something that happened at work? You may be eating to cover up emotions. Realizing you emotionally eat doesn't mean you will stop right away. Recognizing your eating patterns is the first step. There are different levels of awareness. Eventually, you will identify you are not hungry but in fact mad, happy, sad, frustrated, lonely, etc., and you will not reach for food. You will learn to identify your emotions and deal with them in a healthy way.

Distinguishing between physical and emotional hunger can be difficult at first:

04.14.06

Deep down I've known I had a food addiction, but I never paid this much attention to it. I can't believe how messed up my relationship with food is now that I have brought it to the forefront of my consciousness. For example, last Thursday was an exercise day. I had big time PMS. I was tired. I was cranky. I was sore. I sat down on the couch and didn't think I could peel myself off it. It was a nice, sunny day and Chet wanted to walk. I managed to get up and changed into my sweats, and we went for a walk for fifteen or twenty minutes. I walked. I hated every minute. When we came back I was more tired and achy than before we went. My knees hurt a lot that day. We went upstairs to lift weights. I felt like my arms were rubber and I didn't want to try to lift. I talked to Chet and told him I felt that way. I didn't want to lift. I felt guilty that I didn't want to lift. I was hungry.

Now comes the hard part, was I physically hungry or did I want to eat because I felt guilty for not exercising, and feeling bad about eating is easier for me than feeling guilty that I don't exercise enough? Was I physically hungry or was I sore and sad that I was sore? I felt droopy. I thought I was a fat, lazy sack and I would never lose weight again. But... that didn't change the fact that I was physically hungry and I went downstairs and grabbed some food. I went back up to spot Chet while he lifted and I ate. I felt bad about eating. I decided that I was physically hungry, but I felt bad about eating since I wasn't exactly sure if I was eating to feed my addiction. Now, even if I am physically hungry, am I going to feel bad eating since I am not sure if I am eating emotionally or not? I feel like I am crazy. Babies know if they are hungry or not. Why am I having such a hard time figuring it out?

It does get easier the more you practice!

I know I'm not physically hungry. Now what do I do?!

Since your automatic response was to reach for food for a long time, you'll probably find yourself wondering what to do with yourself once you start identifying that you are not physically hungry. I mention throughout this book the different things I found myself doing, but I'm sure you will find what works for you the more you practice.

It will depend on the reasons behind your desire to eat as to what you'd like to do instead of turning to food. For example, if you are stressed out you may want to journal, talk to a friend, or exercise to release pent up energy. If you are bored, you may want to work on one of your favorite hobbies, clean, read a book, or work on a crossword puzzle.

We often have activities or hobbies we enjoy doing, but as life goes on we forget that we enjoyed them. We get busy with family, work, or friends, and find ourselves putting it to the side. For example, I forgot that I enjoy drawing. I like to draw for the sake of drawing. Last year I found myself expressing myself through pictures as well. Sometimes my feelings were so intense and confusing that I would draw a picture of them to get them out of my system.

Instead of eating you can:

- Journal
- Talk to a friend/family member
- Meditate
- Pray
- Read
- Listen to music
- Exercise
- Go for a stroll and enjoy your neighborhood
- Take in a sunset
- Enjoy the flowers
- Watch the birds
- Clean/get organized
- Play a board game
- Watch or play sports

- Practice yoga
- Tap into your creative side: draw, paint, arrange flowers, knit, cross-stich, sing, dance, play music, do origami (paper-folding projects… one of my patients showed me pictures of his modular origami. It is beautiful and keeps your hands busy for hours).
- Pamper yourself: take a bubble bath, get a massage, paint your nails, give yourself a facial
- Use a heating pad to relieve sore muscles or get cozy before bed
- Stretch while watching TV or listening to music.

Practice, practice, practice.

The new behaviors will come faster and faster. Soon it will become automatic.

I wish I could tell you exactly what would soothe you, give you comfort when you need it. However, it is up to you to figure it out. I had a patient tell me that to blow off steam and concentrate on something else he enjoyed welding. Never in a million years would I have come up with that solution! I am not a welder. I don't know anyone who welds. It was a perfect example of how a person needs to think about what they need and look within for the answer. Most of the time you will be the best one to answer that question for yourself.

Susan Albers has a good book you can use as a guide to get more ideas – check out "50 Ways to Soothe Yourself Without Food".

Accept the different levels of awareness.

Realize that each step is an important part of your journey to good health. You can't get to your goal without going through all the steps in between:

1. Acknowledge your problem and admit you need help.

2. Realize that you *ate* for emotional hunger, not physical hunger, after you've eaten.

3. Realize that you *are eating* for emotional hunger, not physical hunger, while you are eating.

4. Realize that you are *about to eat* for emotional hunger, but *you can't seem to stop yourself and you eat anyway.*

5. Realize that you are *about to eat* for emotional hunger, and *you can pause to think* about what is driving your food intake, but you *eat anyway.*

6. Realize that you are *about to eat* for emotional hunger. Y*ou can pause to think* about what is driving your food intake. Y*ou identify your emotional/environmental triggers* and *you stop yourself and do something more positive instead.*

You may find that you feel worse about your food issues after you realize what you are doing to yourself. You won't know how to stop instantaneously. Being more aware of it and not being able to stop it yet can be scary. The different levels of awareness are all part of the process. You will go through each phase until you are able to stop it before it happens. Be kind to yourself as you learn how to change.

If you have a slip up do not beat yourself up and continue in the negative behavior.

You have to shake it off. We can learn from our mistakes and continue to move forward. Every moment is a new beginning. No looking back. Keep practicing.

Sometimes our slip ups are not as bad as we think. Often when we are getting the urge to overeat, it is a signal for us to look past the hunger to find out what we are feeling. We can then acknowledge our feelings and deal with them in a healthy way.

It's a process.

I've been applying these ideas for years and I've gotten stronger, but it has been a struggle. It was like the old way of thinking was fighting with the new way of thinking. The chronic dieter voice inside me was fighting with the nurturing voice. The next chapter contains more journal entries as I worked on this process. It is very clear that my changes didn't happen overnight!

Chapter 10
Trials, Triumphs, and Confusion of this Journey:
Some of my Thoughts along the Way

10.05.05

I HATE it!!!! I really can't stand it ANYMORE!!!! I get down to 265 pounds and jack it up every time. I feel crappy about food more often than not. No matter what book I read or doctor I talk to that tells me I should only eat whole grains, veggies, fruit, and lean protein, I don't want to freakin' do it. How many meals of baked fish or chicken and steamed veggies can I eat? I get totally bored with food. It amazes me. How many Brussel sprouts, asparagus spears, broccoli florets, carrots, celery, cabbage, onions, or kale can I possibly eat? How many flax seed fruit shakes can I drink? I want lasagna, pizza, wings, cake, cookies, pie, etc. I don't want to have to try this hard. I DON'T WANT TO DO IT ANYMORE!!!! Who the heck do you know that eats no refined sugar or flour? Is it true that none of us should be? My brother stopped drinking soda, cut back considerably on beer, only drank water and he lost about 80 pounds in a year. That's all it took? A change in beverages?!!! I lost 70 pounds in two years. That sucks in comparison!!!! I still have almost 100 more to go and that sucks even more. I disgust myself. I feel weak. I am so frickin' fed up.

I am tired. I am tired of trying so hard. I am tired of feeling like I lost control. I am tired of exercising every Tuesday, Thursday, and Sunday. What if I want to do something else? What if I want to sit down? I need to sit down. I need to slow down.

In Virginia I got down to 260 pounds. I moved back to Wilkes-Barre, blinked and gained 35 pounds. I lost another 35 pounds (the same 35 pounds?!) last spring. I gained back about 20 pounds over the summer. I got back down to 265 by the end of summer. I can't seem to break the 260-pound mark and it drives me crazy. I don't know what it is about that weight. I know I start to feel good about myself around this weight. I can start seeing my cheekbones. I start to notice muscles where there weren't any before. I fit into smaller clothes. I think a "such and such" won't hurt (insert your food of choice — this week apple dumpling and donuts). Then I have one, then two and three. Next thing you know I ate one "bad" thing a day for a week, two "bad" things a day for two weeks, etc., and I have gained 20 pounds in a month. It would take me one month to gain it, but four months to lose it and I do it all the damn time. I am SO TIRED. I can't stand it anymore.

I watched a show on TLC last week about the 1000-pound man. It was crazy upsetting to see these super obese people. They had to break down the walls to get the poor guy out. It was so sad. He insisted that he ate no more than a "normal" size person would eat. That can't be true. Does he believe that, or does he just want to? I ate four donuts today throughout the course of the day. Is that "normal"?

I feel like Steve Martin in "Planes, Trains, and Automobiles"...I want some fucking carbs,

right fucking now...a fucking donut, a fucking
candy bar, a fucking potato chip, lots of
carbohydrates and some fat... right fucking now. I
think I will go throw my husband's donuts off the
side of the porch like Frisbees. That ought to
make me feel better.

(Note 12.2.2013: It is interesting for me to read the above entry. I
don't remember weight cycling like that. I don't remember trying to
focus on what foods I ate. Obviously at this point I hadn't given up
on the idea that I *had* to eat "healthy" all the time. I hadn't realized
yet that "healthy" changes all the time. I hadn't given myself
permission to eat whatever I wanted. I do remember being that
frustrated, but I have no recollection of my weight going up and
down as much as 35 pounds so frequently. Another note: one day I
was very angry and went to eat my husband's donuts, and instead I
did end up throwing them off the porch. It did make me feel better.
We may have had chocolate-obsessed squirrels for a while, but it
was worth it!)

03.26.06
        Ok, sure doc, I won't eat whole-wheat pasta
anymore. That's my problem... the whole-wheat pasta.
How about the donuts I had Thursday? The wine I
had Friday night on the phone with Gloria after we
found out that our night shift girl quit? The
shrimp with cheese sauce over regular pasta I had
the next night? How about the cheesecake for
dessert I got when I was full, but since my
friends ordered dessert and said, "come on Jule, I
know how much you like dessert", I said "duh, ok
then give me the cheesecake why don't you"? I
don't know what the heck I'm doing. I keep going
back to my doctor week after week and she asks me
what my problem is, why I think I keep gaining

weight, and I tell her I added whole-wheat pasta.
Yes, pasta is my problem!!! Not peanut butter
cups, coffee, alcohol, cheesecake, donuts, and
more… not those things, it must be that whole-
wheat pasta!!! Who the heck am I kidding?!

I don't know why I am continuing to make bad
decisions every day. It's like since I know I am
going to weigh in on Wednesday, I don't pay
attention on Thursday, Friday, Saturday and Sunday
morning and then I try to make up for it Sunday
afternoon, Monday, Tuesday and Wednesday. That is
not how it works Jule!!! I am making my pancreas
work overtime in the latter half of the week and
then try to make up for it in the early part of
the following week. For all I know the damage has
been done; even if I am not gaining that much
weight, I am going to burn my pancreas cells out
and send myself into full blown diabetes. When I
get diabetes it will be nobody's fault but my own.
I know what I have to do to stay healthy. I am
lucky that I found out what to do when I am young,
but I won't listen to my own advice. If I can't
listen to myself, why do I think this book is
going to matter? Why do I think that other people
will follow my advice if I won't?

I think I need to ask my friends for help. I
asked Chet for help and that didn't do much good.
He is still buying junk food, "hiding" it from me,
but I can find it if I want to, and if he is
eating it after dinner of course I want some too.
I don't even like Oreos, but if he is eating them
I want them. He has been good with exercising with
me and that is a big plus, but somehow I find the
junk food. A couple friends found out that I drive
by Krispy Kreme donuts going to Gram's house every

Wednesday. The last few weeks they have been
giving me money for a dozen and a half. While I am
there, I think I might as well get the other half
dozen to round it out and "give them to Chet".
Yeah, that's it, they are for Chet. Well, I will
eat one in the car on the way home… that won't
hurt. And it is Thursday after all, a week until I
weigh in, so I might as well have a couple donuts
on break with Gloria. Might as well throw in a cup
of coffee while I am at it. IT DOESN'T WORK THAT
WAY JULIE. YOU HAVE TO STOP.

I need help. I think I am going to explain
to my friends that I am behaving in a way that is
not good for my health. Overeating and drinking is
worse for me than it is for them since I have
insulin resistance. Maybe I will explain to them
that I am giving myself diabetes by doing all
these things that I happen to want to do more of
when I am with them. I am not blaming them. It is
my own choice, but if you wave crack in front of
an addict's face they are going to take it from
you and smoke it, even if it is a behavior they
want to stop.

(Note: the above entry shows how a weekly weigh-in, regardless of
who is doing the weighing, may lead to the weekly cycle of
overeating in the early part of the week and restricting in the latter
half of the week. Weighing myself has always messed me up. I'm
messed up enough on my own to keep adding fuel to the fire!)

04.21.06

Last night I didn't know what I wanted to
do. Thursday is usually a hard day since I am
tired by then and don't feel like cooking,
exercising, or doing anything. My knees have been

bothering me so I told Chet I better go buy new sneakers. We went to a couple stores and I couldn't find the style I liked. Then we went out to eat. It should've been an easy night.

I wanted a chicken cheesesteak. Here is how it went in my mind: I caught my reflection in the window and thought 'I can't believe how wide I am and why didn't Chet tell me how huge I look in this T-Shirt?' We open the door and the first thing I do is scan the dining area to see who's there. 'Oh, good, there is a girl that is bigger than me, then maybe people won't stare at me since they are looking at her. I wonder why she is fat… why she overeats… what bothers her?' Then I see a young, thin couple with kids look at me, and I am sure they are thinking what a fat pig I am and that they are hoping their kids don't become fat pigs like me. Then I see some old ladies and wonder if they have had any messed up internal dialog and if, when I am their age, I will still be doing this. Then I see two college guys who are obviously buff and work out all the time. I am embarrassed that they will think I never work out or have any idea how to be healthy. Deep breath…. this is all before I ordered. I wonder what Chet was thinking, probably about what he was going to order.

Then I get around to thinking about what I want for dinner and all I can think is that I can't believe I want a chicken cheesesteak. I should've ordered a salad. Then we sit and, instead of enjoying my husband's company, I continue to scan the room and wonder what these people are thinking. Then I try to convince myself that they are probably more worried about

themselves to give a hoot as to what I ordered and
probably have problems of their own. This kind of
paranoid thinking is egotistical. What makes me
think perfect strangers think anything about me?
As if they have nothing better to think about!

When we finally do get our order I tried to
eat slowly, chew, taste and enjoy my food.
Normally I am done ten minutes before Chet, but we
finished eating at the same time. I was amazed!
The hoagie tasted good and I felt satisfied. I
wonder how much more I could enjoy my food if I am
not scanning the room to see if anyone is looking
at me and wondering what they are thinking.

5.12.06

I figured that since I have this crazy
dialog in my head all the time I might as well
take control of it. Every single time I think
negatively about myself or anything else, I repeat
a positive statement instead until it doesn't
sound so foreign. For example, if I look in the
mirror and think 'I can't believe how huge my
double chin is!', I change it to, 'I'm blessed to
have such pretty eyes, hair, nails, etc'. If I
think negatively about our lack of money, I change
the thought to being thankful for all we have in a
world where so many have so little. It has been
difficult, but not nearly as difficult as feeling
like a piece of crap for overeating and for my
weight. It is MUCH, MUCH harder to feel terrible
about eating than to feel or express the actual
feeling you are trying to forget by overeating. It
is a relief to tell my husband how I feel about
something than to hold it in, overeat, and feel
worthless. It feels better for me to tell my boss

if I feel overworked and ask for help instead of shoving my face at work, sucking it up, and driving myself into the ground. It feels better to admit I am too tired to drive up to Scranton to sit with Gram, and instead I rest, and go up over the weekend. That's better than pushing myself, feeling worse, and eating to "feel better". It is healthier for me to tell my husband I need some friend time, let him do his studying, take off to Philly, and feel better, instead of sitting home, getting cranky with Chet, and sitting on the couch and eating all night. It is amazing how much is going on in my head and my heart. I had to learn to listen a little harder. Ok, a lot harder.

5.26.06

Last week I watched a talk show with anorexic people. It was extremely sad. Their bones were sticking out. They were sitting on the stage lying about the fact that they have been eating more when it is painfully obvious they were not. Then it dawned on me that they have the same problem with food and themselves that I do, only on the opposite end of the spectrum. I've heard sexuality explained on a spectrum before, so why not food relationships?

If these eating disorders are all deviations from the norm, why is it that the overweight are not treated with the same compassion and empathy as the overly thin? Many people would look at the anorexic person and feel bad for them that this terrible disease made them sick. Many people would look at me or any other overweight person and get disgusted that we "let ourselves go" or "have no self-control". Being on either end of the food spectrum can have devastating effects on your physical health, self-esteem, and your relationships. The public needs education on eating disorders so that they can support the people in their lives who are afflicted by them.

Last night was Chet's graduation. I was incredibly proud of him. How did we celebrate? You guessed it... we had family and friends over for cake. Food. Later in the evening I was upset that I didn't remember finishing my cake. I remember the first few bites were heavenly, chocolate cake, chocolate icing, and chocolate pudding in the middle. That's all I remembered... the first few bites. I was doing well with being conscious of my eating and I got upset that I didn't remember eating the rest. Then I cleaned off the table and saw half of my cake was on my plate. That was why I didn't remember eating it! I was really excited!!! Last night I thought about whether I was hungry, decided I was, and finished my cake without feeling bad at all. Amazing!

8.7.06

Here's the thing.... for the last several months I haven't written in my journal or my book. I haven't been thinking about food. I finally allowed myself to weigh what I weigh and eat what I want to eat. I didn't have the usual junk to write about. Since I haven't been weighing myself I don't feel like I am exactly sure how my progress is, but my clothes are fitting about the same so I'm sure I'm fine. It is quite remarkable that in the past several months I haven't gained weight, even though I am not paying too close attention to my diet. That has never been the case with me!!! I've always obsessed about every calorie, gram of fat, or carb to stay the same or lose weight. That's because I've had the desire to shove my face with a range of different foods for a range of different reasons, unknown to me at the time (hence the nature of addiction).

Over the last several months I've learned a lot about physical hunger and physically feeling full. I've learned when I am tired that it's OK to take a nap. I also learned that sometimes I'm tired because I haven't exercised in a while, so I'd better go get the blood pumping. I've learned to pay attention to my body. Guess what I was forgetting to pay attention to... my mind. I was used to filling my brain with obsessive thoughts about food, guilt, more food, calories, fat, carbs, protein, fiber, feeling fat, worthless, ugly, etc., that when I stopped filling my brain with those things I didn't know what else to do with my brain. I started to fill it up with different scenarios for the future and thinking about the past. I continued with the obsessive thinking, only now it wasn't about food... it was about my relationship, my family's relationship with food and how they got that way, anyone I know and their history with depression, how everyone has a vice, how I didn't think I would be working where I am working, how I'm not using my degree, how I should be making more money, how I never have enough time to do anything I want... all my fears came to the surface too... how I'm afraid deep down that Chet is going to die way before me, how I may have to deal with his old age at the same time as my parents and some of my friends (two of my best friends are also twenty years

older than me), how I may want to get pregnant
even though I've spent most of my life telling
myself I didn't since I think I'm infertile (At a
young age I knew I didn't get periods like I
should and it probably meant I wouldn't be able to
have kids.), how I should get pregnant sooner
rather than later because of our age difference,
how I feel like I should go back to school but I
don't like how the last seven years either Chet or
I have been in school — it's difficult having a
full time student in the house, for both
people.... There is more floating up in there —
it's like 'shut the f#$% up already!'

Since I stopped thinking about food and my
weight it was like there was a void in my brain. I
didn't use food to make me stop thinking
obsessively about everything in my life. I didn't
know how to cope with any of the feelings that
started to creep into my brain that now filled the
space that was previously reserved for negative
food thought. What I need to do is start quieting
my mind. It's ironic that I made up a fake Tai Chi
workout at work to help me cope with my day. It
started as a joke, but I started thinking I should
try it. I borrowed a DVD from my friend this
weekend and I like it. I am going to try to get
back into meditation. I need to start talking to
my friends earlier than when I am about to freak
out about something. I don't think I would have
talked today if one of my friends didn't ask me
what was wrong. I don't think I knew until she
asked. I need to start talking to everyone a lot
more than I do. Part of my problem is that I often
feel guilty for feeling the way I do.

Instead of forgiving myself since I'm only human, I obsess about it. I Googled the official term... I'm a ruminator, an over-thinker. This is ironic since another definition is the chronic regurgitation, chewing, and re-swallowing of previously ingested food. It all comes back to food for me, doesn't it?!

2.28.07

I've been thinking about how several circumstances in the last few weeks have brought back a whole flood of old feelings. Feelings that I tried to bury for a long time and tried to ignore. I never got a chance to process and heal from those feelings. Reading Rethinking Thin, talking about eating disorders in class, and going for counseling has brought up a whole lot that I hadn't bothered to deal with or bring to the surface... a lot of the things I tried to eat away.

A major shift in my self-image came around four years ago when I realized I had a serious problem with food. I hurt for a long time, but I hadn't paid much attention to it. Since I was six I felt out of place. I got picked on. I didn't look like my friends. The guilt started young in regards to eating. I remember being eight years old and buying candy with my friends and feeling terrible after I ate it since I knew it made me fatter.

I always had friends, but I felt like nobody understood my pain. I felt like nobody understood how hard it was to be unable to run around and play like everyone else. I couldn't try out for cheering or sports like my friends. I couldn't do

a pull-up for gym glass. I couldn't hang upside
down on the monkey bars. I didn't have boys
talking to me. In middle school I was paranoid how
big my butt looked when I was bowling. I had a
terrible time climbing the steps in between class
in middle school and high school. In college when
I was thinner and in better shape, I could still
barely make it to the third floor without being
out of breath. It hurt every time I couldn't
buckle my seatbelt or fit into a desk or a booth
at a restaurant. I got embarrassed every time I
lost weight and gained it back. If I talked to
someone whom I hadn't seen for a long time, I
barely heard what they said. I only worried about
what they thought about the weight I gained.
Trying on clothes, no matter if it was a plus size
shop or not, was a terrible experience. I would
get frustrated because nothing fit right or looked
good on me, and I often left the store with a
bigger size than I thought I would need. It hurt
every time I walked or ran for exercise and people
yelled derogatory things at me out of their car
windows or from their front porch. I felt like I
let people down every time I gained weight because
I felt like people expected me to know better. It
hurt that I could never go to my friend's pool and
feel comfortable. It took me 20 years to go into a
pool without a T-shirt on to cover up. It
embarrassed me when I could barely lift my butt
out of the pool when we were done. It hurt when
Chet couldn't get his arms around me to hug me. It
hurt when I couldn't stand for a long time, like
in lab or at work, without pain in my feet, knees,
legs, and hips. I was sad every time I had to come
home and sleep because I was too tired to do

anything else and I had to ice half my body to
help to reduce the inflammation. It hurt when I
twisted my ankle several times because I couldn't
help but think it was my weight that crushed it.
It still hurts when I barely fit into the desk. It
hurts when I look at other people that I know who
are hurting for the same reasons I hurt in the
past. It hurts when people in my classes make
references to the lazy obese people that you'd
think would know enough when to stop eating. Is
that what they thought of me? It hurt every single
time a doctor saw nothing but my fat.... every
time they told me all my problems were from
overeating, even if I told them I couldn't stop.
It hurt when I had to take time off from graduate
school. It hurt when I didn't go to my graduation
because I wasn't proud of myself and didn't want
to find out whether or not I could fit into a
gown. It hurt that we didn't have our wedding the
first time we said we would since I felt bad about
how fat I was. I hurt myself by not sharing with
people... not letting them know how I felt.

It hurts that I never give myself a break.

It hurts that I never give myself credit for my
accomplishments.

It hurts that I'm still not sure how to stop
hurting myself.

3.1.07

    I am supposedly writing a book about how I've conquered emotional eating despite my insulin resistance. However, I only seem to record all the negative. How am I supposed to show people how I've changed if I haven't recorded it along the way? I should start pointing out the good things I've achieved.

    If you take a snapshot of me, more specifically my thought patterns, two years ago, the only thing I focused on was food and how I looked to other people. I spent the majority of my day adding up calories, fat, protein, carbs, fiber, etc. I weighed myself several times a day and felt worthless when the scale didn't say what I thought it should. I worried that my appearance disgusted other people. If I went out to eat I'd have this mental dialogue: 'you shouldn't be eating restaurant food, shouldn't be eating dessert, shouldn't be drinking that, shouldn't be eating that much in one sitting'… and on and on….. and on and on and on. It was all I could do to try to pay attention to the conversation in between. I'd wonder if anyone added up how much I ate, or if other people in the restaurant noticed I ordered something fried or added sugar to my iced tea.

    If you took another snapshot of me today, you would have a hard time believing that I was the same person. I ordered lunch without one thought of the nutritional content of the food, or if anyone else wondered if I should be eating that. When looking at the menu the only thoughts going through my head were if I would enjoy eating what I ordered and if my body would feel ok after I ate it. Who would have thought that one year prior I had such a hard time ordering from a menu? Or that I practically had an anxiety attack every time I was around food and people simultaneously? Or that I wasted valuable brainpower on negative self-talk and caloric intake?

Here I sit in my buddy's lab writing. I've gone from having a panic attack when walking into the Chem building, to feeling good enough to meet everyone he works with and not have one single thought about how I looked, or if they thought I was intelligent enough to be in their space. It is amazing.

How did this great transformation take place? Did I wake up one day and years of negative self-talk and its' impact on my self-esteem disappear? No. Was it easy? No. It happened over time. Can you do it too? Yes!

It all started when I stopped weighing myself. It took a lot of restraint to stay off the scale. It was like a meter to tell me how I felt. When you've used the scale every day, many times a day, for years and years to tell you how you felt about yourself, it can be a hard thing to stop doing. Recording your weight can be a hard habit to break, especially when you have charts with your poundage and measurements on it, some of them dating back as far as fourth grade. It's not like I would only weigh myself on my own scale. For a while I couldn't walk past any scale without hopping on it- my parents, my Gramma's, my friends', etc. Any scale I would see would call me over to it. For a while it almost felt like I would have some sort of fit walking past a scale.

'Come on Jule... you know you need to know how you feel about yourself. Step right up!' At my parents' house I would go upstairs and walk past their scale in the hallway itching to jump on. Some of my friends have theirs in their bathrooms and it was all I could do, like it took every fiber in my being, not to get on...Gained a pound? 'Yep, just as I thought... I'm a loser.' Sunny outside... in a good mood... before I enjoy myself, let me get on the scale to determine my worth... gained a pound? 'Gee, all of a sudden it looks like rain, doesn't it?' Lost a pound today... 'Well, I guess I can continue smiling since at least I am doing something right.' Later the same afternoon, back to the same weight... 'see, I guess I had lost a lot of water weight overnight and now I gained a pound so I'd better go beat myself up. Guess I'm not worthy to smile after all'. Tell you what, after I made my husband hide our scale it was a little weird for me to realize that I would have to pay attention to my real mood and not the one dictated by the scale. Hmmm... I woke up and I'm not sure how I feel... where is my scale (mood meter)? Downstairs. Shoot, I don't know where Chet put it. Should I go look? I don't have time for that.

'How do I feel today?' I'd have to ask myself. Well, for weeks my answer was fat. Then I realized what many people have said before, fat is not a feeling — it's an adjective or a noun. I happen to have extra fat on my body... I am fat, but I'm also tall, with brown hair, hazel eyes, intelligent ... true is true. Then, I started to ask myself what I was besides fat. 'Hmm... fat, yes, I've previously established that, fat and....

fun, smart, pretty, loving... etc.' It got easier the more I did it. I started to tap into my heart, and every day I came up with new emotions and positive adjectives for myself.

It seems like a lot of work. Who goes around praising themselves all day? Who has time to build themselves up every day? Well, I certainly had enough time to add up my nutritional information, weigh myself and beat myself up all the time, so I must have the time to build myself up. I told myself over and over... if you have used all that time for negative, you can use all that time for positive. Ultimately, it's nobody's choice but our own.

Once I got used to not weighing myself I began to concentrate on how my body felt. Did I have a lot of energy today and could workout hard? Was my energy a little low? Should I do a ten-minute warm up to see how my body would respond? If I felt better after ten minutes I would up the exercise intensity level. If I felt crappy I would cut it short and stretch well and meditate. I started to respect my body. As the days went by I felt stronger and healthier. The stronger I felt, the less what I looked like mattered. Sure, someday I would like to be thinner for many different reasons, but I am more fit now than I've been in seven years. I've been doing Tae Bo for at least six months and my entire body has more muscle mass. I feel good, so I look good. I feel I look good, so I look even better. It's all about how I feel — it finally has nothing at all to do with what my scale, my mood meter, reads.

Exercise wasn't the only thing that changed when I started listening to my body. My relationship with food changed dramatically as well. A couple years ago I gave myself permission to eat whatever I wanted. First I craved all junk food that I hadn't allowed myself to eat for a long time. Then, after I ate junk I started listening to how my body felt after I ate. When I eat junk I feel like junk... go figure. Now, if I think about eating ice cream, I can eat one serving or even a half of a serving, eat it slowly and enjoy how it tastes. I've learned that snacking will keep me from feeling deprived. I don't hide the fact that I ate something. I don't jump on the scale as soon as I'm done eating. I don't immediately go out and walk for an hour because of the guilt. The key is now I don't overeat. I eat when I'm hungry and stop when I am satisfied. I don't feel guilty about anything I put in my mouth. There was a time when I could have rambled off everything I put into my mouth for at least a week — maybe longer. Now I barely remember what I ate yesterday, let alone how many calories I ate. Listening to how my body feels after I eat helps me make better choices for myself in the future. I know if I eat a whole tub of peanut butter and chocolate candy I will most likely have a stomachache afterwards. I know I will feel like blah and I won't want to move at all- so exercise is out. I'm not saying I don't ever eat "junk" but the majority of the foods (85-90%) are healthy — whole grains, lean meats, fruits, veggies, and plenty of water. That good fuel makes my whole body feel better. I can exercise harder, think more clearly, and sleep better, and I end up feeling better about myself overall. Why would you choose food that makes your

body feel like crap, when you can choose to fuel
your body with good food for maximum energy
instead? Yes, I know the answer… because some of
that junk tastes so damn good! But… a little bit
of the "junk" will probably not make my body feel
bad, whereas a lot of the "junk" will. I have
found the balance and my body and mind is better
for it.

6.6.07

    The past year has been great. I've done
something that I've NEVER done in the past. I've
stayed at the same weight! That was my goal... to
not be on any specific "diet", try to eat mostly
nutritionally dense food, be comfortable with my
body, regardless of my weight, and most
importantly not let food control my life. I did
it! I am very proud of myself. Now what?

    Well, now I want to lose weight. I know I'm
healthier than ever, but I could improve. I don't
want to be a beanpole; I do want to keep feeling
more fit. I can exercise several times a week, go
for three-hour hikes, paint my aunt's house, push
Gram around in her wheelchair for a couple miles,
and clean all day. I know I'm in good shape. I
can't imagine all I could do if I lost another 20,
50, or 80 pounds. Can I imagine being lighter,
healthier, and more fit? I think the problem is
that I can't. I felt unhealthy and unfit for so
long that I think I expected to not be able to
change. I'm happy to do what I can do now. I
should be happy, and I am, but I'm also
complacent. Sigh.

My PCOS symptoms have all but disappeared. I have regular periods as long as I am using my progesterone cream, my acne has decreased considerably, and my hormone levels are all within normal limits. Shoot. Now I don't have anything to hide behind. Before I could blame my weight on hormonal imbalances. Well, now I am not as imbalanced. Now I have no excuse. Now I have to try to lose weight.

I feared that if I paid attention to my food intake again it would become an obsession. I feared I would go back to adding up my calories, grams of carbs, fat, protein, fiber, etc. in my head all day and not have the ability to focus on anything else. I feared that I wouldn't lose any more weight. After all, I have been extremely comfortable eating what I have been eating this past year... I don't want to feel like I'm not getting enough food. How much food is enough? I know I do a better job of not shoveling it, but maybe I could pay more attention.

(Note 12.2.2013: When I think about "watching" what I eat, I start to lose control again, or at least I feel like I do. This next entry makes an interesting point. It is just one week later.)

6.12.07

Last week I called a friend to tell him I was back at it again... I was shoving my face. He asked me how bad it was and I told him it was awful. He asked if I was eating a dozen donuts or a whole cake or anything and I told him no. Hmm.... maybe it wasn't as bad as I thought.

When I thought about it, I knew I wasn't exactly choosing nutrient-dense foods, but I wasn't exactly going off the deep end either. Ok, so I had cake and ice cream one day for dinner. I only had one serving of each, so it wasn't like I was sitting watching TV with a feedbag around my neck. I ate it. I enjoyed it. Then it was over. I didn't go back for more. I didn't stop at the store on the way home to stock up on junk food. I didn't have any fiber or protein with dinner for one day... so what! Compared to what I used to do, these last couple weeks were mild. What hit me was that I felt so out of control! I had plenty of control, but I still felt like I was spinning faster and faster. At least I knew enough this time to talk about it.

I have made a lot of changes lately... I left a job I wasn't happy with, I decided to go back to school this Fall and not wait another year like I originally planned, and I decided to take the Summer off to finish my book before going back to school. All these negative thoughts were going through my head: How would we afford our expenses if I didn't work for a while? Would we be able to pay off our student loans? You know what happened the last time you tried graduate school, would you be able to keep up? What if you got sick again? Asking your family to help you out is a big deal, should you bother them? Do you think anyone is going to read your book anyway? The signal for me to stop and take a good look at how all this made me feel was noticing the poor food choices I made and the lack of desire to exercise lately.

I felt like I was at square one. Then I realized that was ridiculous. I learned a lot over the last five years and there was no way it could all be erased with a piece of cake and a scoop of ice cream! I have done the hard work. I am the healthiest I've ever been, physically and emotionally. There is nowhere to go but up because I refuse to go back!

Today my husband and I stopped for lunch while we were out running errands. We stopped at a fast food restaurant. I had a cheeseburger, chocolate milk and good conversation and went on with my day. In the past, I would have practically had a panic attack if someone wanted fast food. I would have run down their whole menu, realizing that there were more healthful things I could be eating at home. I would have worried about what the person taking my order would have thought when I said all I wanted was a junior cheeseburger. I would have had this whole dialog going in my head of what everyone else was thinking... 'Yeah, right. *She* only wants a junior cheeseburger. Why doesn't she get the other cheeseburger and extra, extra-large fry with that to go with her extra, extra wide rear end like she wants to? I bet she'll take that to go... to go with the family size bag of chips she's got at home.' I would have been too embarrassed to order, then I would have been too embarrassed to sit down and eat, and I would have thought everyone stared at me to see if I would go back for more. I wouldn't have enjoyed any of my food and my skin would have been crawling. Then I would have gotten mad at present company for "forcing" me to go to a fast food restaurant. I would have been miserable for the rest of the day. I would have thought about it for days. I would have wasted valuable energy over a freakin' cheeseburger. No more!

I used to have dialog like that ALL THE TIME in my head. I wouldn't go anywhere (restaurants, grocery stores, malls, etc.) without thinking about what other people were probably thinking about me. The grocery store was the worst. I used to think other people were looking in my cart and giving me a 'tsk, tsk' in their heads. I used to look for the most non-judgmental-looking checker. What does a non-judgmental-looking checker look like you ask? A fellow fatty of course! Man, that was quite judgmental of *me*, wasn't it? What a hypocrite! It's amazing that I don't do that at all anymore. I never worry about anything I put in my cart. I feel fine putting my ice cream next to my cottage cheese or my candy bar next to my whole grain cereal. I know I eat mostly nutrient-dense food, food that makes my body feel good, and that's all that matters.

I have gotten rid of the "good" food and "bad" food idea. I didn't think it would be possible. I don't know if people believe me when I tell them, but my courses in biochemistry helped me figure this one out. The reactions I studied tell me that the carbon, hydrogen, oxygen and nitrogen from our food goes through the same metabolic reactions in our bodies, regardless of the source. An apple or a cookie will get broken down for energy if your body needs fuel. Physical hunger is a sign that we need fuel. Anything I eat can turn into energy. The cookie isn't a "bad" food. If I am hungry my body will burn it for fuel just like the apple would. However, all food can also turn into fat... a cookie and an apple can be broken down and get fed through reactions that build fat molecules for storage. So, there are no

magical lists of foods that can keep me skinny.
The "magic" comes from tapping into what your body
is telling you it needs.

I used to practically hear the food calling
me. 'Julie, you know I'm in the freezer, don't
you? Why haven't you eaten me yet?' I would hold
off as long as I could and then I'd end up eating
the whole pint of ice cream. I don't do that at
all anymore. I wait until the next time I am
physically hungry and then I will have one serving
of whatever "bad" food I'm craving. For example, I
bought these little ice cream bites a couple
months ago. I would eat one or two at a time (a
serving was five) after a meal if I wanted
something sweet and pineapple wasn't gonna cut it.
Today I went to put my frozen veggies away in our
big freezer and saw the ice cream bites on the
door. I couldn't believe I never finished them
off! I didn't even want them anymore. I showed
Chet. He and I were amazed. Several years ago they
would have been gone a week after purchase at
most. [6.15.08 I reread this entry and realized
that I threw out the rest of those ice cream bites
a year later! They were lost and freezer burnt...
obviously they weren't able to "call" me anymore!]

Something I need to work on is giving myself
more credit. I have made huge lifestyle changes
that are going to make me a better, healthier
person for the rest of my life. I am proud but I
need to work on how easily I can forget.

Journaling has helped me. Since my behavior
and attitude towards many different situations
have changed dramatically it is great to flip back
on occasion and see how far I've come.

6.24.07

    I have a lot of people I love. I want to spend time with all of them and help them with whatever they need because of my love for them. I've been off work for three weeks and I've been running all over the place. I've painted over at my aunt's house a couple days, Gramma-sat a couple times a week, gone to family dinners and parties, and helped a friend move several times. I'm tired. I feel like I've been pulled in many different directions.

    My father called me to ask if I was going to sit with my mom while he had his sinus polyps removed. It's outpatient, noninvasive surgery. Since he had gallbladder, foot surgery, and knee surgery all within the last five years, I thought that this was minor in comparison. The thought hadn't crossed my mind to spend the day with him and Mom. Instead of saying yes like I normally would have, I thought about it and knew it wasn't in my heart to do so. I explained to him that I had just gotten home from five days in Philly. I will be in Scranton two days this week to Gramma-sit and a third day this week isn't in the cards for me. I need time for myself. I need time to write. I've been working hard and I'm tired. I felt bad for telling Dad no. In the past I would have eaten since I felt bad. Then I would have gone up to Scranton anyway and not done what I wanted to do. Then I would have eaten more since I would have felt pulled in two million directions. I felt good about not eating. I still felt tired. The only thing I wanted to do was to cook a nice meal with Chet, eat slowly and relax, chill out and have a coffee, take a nap, watch my favorite show and meditate. Then I wanted to work on my book. I took several hours and did exactly what I wanted to do. Now I feel refreshed. I know I will continue to work hard this week and I know I will have the energy to do it. I keep reminding myself that there is nothing wrong with taking care of myself. If I am not fully charged I will not be able to give anything to anyone else like I want to. Many of us feel guilty about feeling like we are letting people down. Since we don't know how to deal with that guilt, we eat. Tonight I thought of what I needed and I gave myself that instead.

I didn't shove my face. I feel healthy and strong. It takes a conscious effort but I am in a better place. I am thankful and peaceful.

(Note: Taking time for myself and giving myself what I need has proven to be quite difficult over the years. I have gotten better at it, but giving too much to others at my expense has been a difficult habit to break. I know a lot of people do this.)

7.15.07

Yesterday I hung out with the guys for the first time in a long time. It was good to see everybody. They seem to be doing well. Seem to be.... I wonder how they truly feel. I wonder if they knew how I felt? I wonder if they knew all those years in that house how terrible I felt about myself? Did they know the negative thought processes I had in my head day in and day out? Did they know I felt out of place all the time? Did they know that I was torn between wanting to be one of the guys and feeling terrible because I was one of the guys? I never felt feminine. I never felt truly happy. All I did was beat myself up all the time.

It's amazing how people you've had in your life can act like a mirror for you. Sometimes to appreciate how you've changed you need to remember how you felt in the past. Once I got over thinking about all that stuff, I settled in and started to listen to their conversations. Part of not feeling like one of the guys was how I never knew all of their inside jokes. I know they've known each other for a long time and I used to feel like an outsider. I think that's why I used to get upset when they would lock me out since I often felt locked out anyway. It had nothing to do with them.... I didn't feel like I was good at being a girl and I obviously wasn't one of the guys. I felt stuck in limbo.

It was nice to see everything in a different light. It was nice to sit back and see how happy they were while reminiscing. They have a lot of funny stories and if I asked them to elaborate they were more than happy to. They have a beautiful thing. You can tell they all love each other. I felt like an idiot because I underestimated how much they loved me too. My self-esteem was so low that I used to feel like they only had me around since I happened to live next to one of them. It took me until I was 29 to realize they had me there because they love me.

At the party I listened to one of their Dad's talk about how the guys saw me in high school. He said I was so inspiring to everyone, including all the parents. He reminded me what an amazing thing I had done. It takes a strong will to start running at 260 pounds at 17 years old and he said "even more balls to join a team knowing damn well I was usually going to be absolutely last". People often told me I was inspiring. When my eating got out of control I felt like such a failure. How inspiring is it to get so fat that you can't run and you go shove donuts down your throat? How inspiring was it that I felt out of control and like there was nothing I could do about it? How inspiring was it that I stopped talking to virtually everyone that cared about me and withdrew into myself? How inspiring was it that I went from smiling all the time senior year of high school to crying every day for years? I felt like a failure for a long time.

Guess what I learned? Everyone messes up sometimes. If you're lucky you have people in your life who will love you anyway. I also learned that I am a strong person for digging myself out of my hole. Maybe I can be an inspiration to others again someday soon. Maybe I am already.

Another cool thing happened at the restaurant when we went out for wings and beer. I didn't have a single negative self-image thought! I didn't add up my calories in my head, or wonder if the guys were wondering how I got so fat or if I should be eating that wing. I paid attention to the conversation and didn't worry about me at all. I realized I didn't cringe when they hugged me, since I didn't care that they knew my girth had grown over the years. I was happy to be around them... I was just me. I don't feel like everything is swirling around me and there is nothing I can do about it. I never feel like I use food as a drug anymore. I never feel that anger and self-hate down in the pit of my stomach. I feel in control. I feel free.

7.27.07

This summer I accomplished a lot. I worked on my book and almost have a first draft complete. I've exercised 6 days a week, including weight training, Tae Bo, hiking, and bike riding. I've eaten healthful foods. I've helped out with Gram. I've spent time with friends and family. However, I always have this feeling deep down that it is not enough... that I am not enough.

I have corrected my behavior and attitude towards food, but I have not gotten rid of the guilt inside me. I feel like I should be doing more... like I should be doing better. I feel like I spread myself too thin, but it doesn't stop me from cramming as much as I can into the day. I make all these goals in my head for the day *all day.* For example, today I was tired. I wanted to chill. Earlier this week I read all of my journal entries from the last four years so I could start adding them into my book and was overwhelmed by the flood of emotions I experienced. On top of that I had a mentally exhausting day with Gram yesterday and I exercised eleven days in a row. I needed to recharge but I kept thinking about what I should be doing instead. I felt like I should clean and organize my house, go through my clothes for work and school, have Mom take my pants in, gather the stuff I want to take to Salvation Army, make plans for vacation, check on my loans for school, exercise, write, read, and edit my book, catch up with my friends, cook, grocery shop,

etc., etc., etc. All day I kept going through what
I should be doing. All day I should have been
relaxing and I didn't. All I did today was paint
my nails, make a nice dinner, watch TV and talk to
my friends, but the whole time I had this guilty
feeling gnawing at my insides. I hate when I am
tired. I was tired all day. I didn't recharge. I
do it to myself. It's insane.

I haven't been employed the last two months,
but I've been working harder than ever. I've been
working on getting as strong as possible, mentally
and physically, before I go back to school. I am
stronger than I've ever been, so why can't I just
chill out? What is this guilt all about? Don't get
me wrong, I have been enjoying myself and I've
felt positive most of the time, but if I could get
rid of this guilt, I'm sure I would enjoy life
even more. I'm not sure how to do that.

9.05.07

As I drove to school on the first day I was
overwhelmed with joy and had to fight back the
tears.... I couldn't ruin my makeup. I was more
nervous than I thought I'd be. I felt much older
than all of the kids. It was clear that I was
bigger than everyone else, but it didn't occur to
me until I sat in my seat and my stomach hit the
desk. Immediately in my own mind I ballooned up to
350 pounds. I got paranoid. I looked around the
room to see who noticed. I felt flushed. I was
embarrassed. Then I realized that my next thoughts
would be to doubt that it was a good idea to go
back to school and to wonder why I thought I could
do it anyway since I am stupid. Then I thought of
a scene in a popular movie and saw myself slapping

myself in the face and yelling, "snap out of it".
I looked down and realized I hadn't suddenly
gained 90 pounds back and my stomach barely
touched the desk and wasn't spilling over it like
I thought. Then I looked around the room and saw a
bunch of nervous faces. I realized they were all
nervous, possibly even more than me. I've had life
experience and formal education and I was
absolutely prepared for the upcoming workload. I
identified my feelings as a mixture of excitement,
happiness, nervousness, and a little anxiety and
gave myself permission to feel those feelings. I
had conversations with some of my loved ones about
those feelings, especially the nervousness and
anxiety. I didn't reach for food since those
feelings came across as feelings and not hunger.

I realize that a year or two ago that
negative self-talk would have continued to
snowball until I couldn't pay attention to a word
my professor said. Then as a "solution" I'd go out
to the nearest vending machine and buy one or more
sweet treats to soothe my pain. It's taken a lot
of hard work but I'm far from that. I know I still
have work to do and eventually I won't need those
"snap out of it" moments because my train of
thought will stop going in that direction all
together.

My life did not necessarily get easier, but I learned how to
handle the cards I was dealt in healthier ways. The next chapter
focuses on one of my biggest coping mechanisms... the Safety Net,
the network of people I have in my life who support me.

Chapter 11
Seek Out Support

The Safety Net

When I went through a hard time last year a loved one gave me the analogy of the safety net. He told me to picture everyone who loves me under me, supporting me and not letting me fall. My closest friends were right under me, giving me the most support. Others were slightly farther away from the center, but lending that extra, needed support. Some friends and family I'd lean on daily. Some a few times a week. Others maybe monthly. Having all those ears to bend did help. Many people didn't know what to say, but most of the time I didn't need them to say anything. I needed them to be there with me, either in person or over the phone. I'd get a card occasionally from a friend and that helped me feel that net stretch out even farther... knowing people were sending me all those thoughts and prayers helped. I'm blessed to have a big safety net, but I truly didn't understand how strong it was until I needed to use it.

You can start building the net so you can use it. The next time you need it, it will be there for you, waiting for you to bounce around in it. One of the good things about building your net is that when those people who supported you through tough times need support themselves, you can be there for them too. Maybe they've learned how to build one by watching you do it.

We all have times in our lives that seem dark, even if we don't have a tendency towards depression. Bad things happen... loved ones get ill or pass away, jobs are lost, money can be tight and relationships end. We are all exposed to difficult situations. In those dark times, it makes it easier to have as much support as possible. If you are lucky, you have people in your life you can lean on. If you are luckier, you know how to lean on them.

I always knew I had a lot of people who loved me. I also felt, for whatever reason, I was the one who was supposed to be strong for everyone else. I thought that somehow it was my job to protect everyone I loved, and sometimes that meant protecting them from feeling bad for me. It is a theme I have found when talking with my patients. Many people who are caregivers by nature feel it is their job to bear the burden of other people's pain, but keep their pain to themselves. People like that often suppress their feelings, and one way to do that is to distract themselves with food.

If you don't have a good support system, make it a priority to build one. If you have friends and don't lean on them, start doing it. Be specific in what you need. For example, someone I know was in the hospital, feeling like nobody cared as she laid there frustrated with her life, crying and wondering why nobody was there to hand her a tissue. I asked if she let her loved ones know how she felt and if she asked for them to come visit. The answer was no. The people who love you cannot read your mind. If you don't ask for what you need, you'll never get it. If you do ask, you may not always get it, but it will never happen if you don't speak up. If someone cannot be there for you the way you need them to be it will hurt, but then maybe you can ask someone else. You won't be able to be there for everyone you care about either. That was something that often bothered me, and to some extent it still does. However, if you have a lot of people in your life it is impossible to support everyone the way you would like to every single time they need you. You will end up letting people down, just like you've been let down. That doesn't mean that both people in the relationship don't care about one another.

Building Relationships and Working on the Ones You've Got

I knew for a long time that I longed for my parents to tell me they loved me. I heard some of my friends' parents tell them. I wished I had that kind of relationship with mine. It bothered me for years. I knew they didn't grow up with their parents telling them, so I knew they were unaccustomed to it. I knew they loved me. I felt it, but sometimes it is nice to hear. That said, it is uncomfortable to say if you've never said it.

My Gram was the first person to whom I said "I love you". She was sick and in the hospital when I was a sophomore in high school. I was close to her. If I lost her and I didn't tell her I loved her I knew I'd regret it. I regretted not telling my other grandparents before they passed away. I wasn't going to let my last opportunity with a grandparent pass by. Ok, I tend to be dramatic... she was only in for gallbladder surgery. She probably wasn't going to pass away anytime soon, but it got me thinking. I made sure to tell her before she went in for her procedure. Guess what happened... she said it back! It felt fantastic.

For quite some time Gram was the only person I said it to on a regular basis. I started to tell my friends on occasion. I held out on telling my parents. I wished they said it to me first. Eventually I decided that nobody taught them, so if it was something I wanted and needed I had better teach them how. One day when leaving their house, I kinda yelled it from the doorway. I'm not sure if they said it back or not, but it was good enough to get me started. I started ending my phone calls that way and they responded with an 'I love you' back. Now, in my mid-thirties, I finally have the thing I always wanted... for them to say it first, without prompting. It feels good.

I started telling everyone in my family after that on occasion. It is always met with an "I love you" in return. One time Mom replied, "tolerate you" … it was funny. Sarcasm does run deep in our family. But yes, sometimes love is tolerating the other person, isn't it?! To know someone and love them anyway… to accept their flaws along with all their good qualities. That's real love. That is also what we need to learn to do for ourselves… to love and accept ourselves.

I felt like all of this "I love you" stuff opened doors. Since my family could handle a verbal expression of loving feelings, I hoped they could listen about how I feel in general. I thought maybe I didn't have to "protect" them anymore from the negative feelings. I've ended up sharing more of everything with them. My concerns, fear or sadness is usually met with the comfort and validation I want and need. It was a tough road, but the results have been priceless.

Letting people know you love them feels good. Getting love in return feels even better. Talking with that patient who was upset about not having anyone there, we ended up discussing the people she had in her life who she knew loved her. The list was quite long. When we got done thinking about all that love, she felt better just knowing they loved her even though they were not present. Her day seemed a little bit brighter.

When you discover how out of control your behavior is, it can be quite overwhelming. Support from friends or outside sources is crucial to helping you along in your journey. You may be surprised when you start talking about how your relationship with food has affected your life, how many others respond by saying they know exactly how you feel. Your journey will be difficult enough without allowing yourself to feel like you are all alone in your battle. If you are uncomfortable sharing with your loved ones initially, support groups can be a great way to get the understanding you need. Some groups probably have meetings in your area. Others meet online in chat rooms or have postings on bulletin boards.

It could be problematic that for a long time you shut people out. People with addictions often keep to themselves. It is ironic, since what they often long for is a connection with something. They pick the substance or activity they are abusing instead of people. I've read that it is because the object or activity won't let them down. Food, gambling, alcohol, sex, shopping, etc., is all predictable. It will ALWAYS produce that high you are looking for or that false feeling of control over your life. I didn't speak with some of my friends for years. I talked with a few, but I never shared my true feelings. I wasn't there for them either. I was lucky to have people who understood and would take me back. You may have done permanent damage to some of your relationships. However, when you are ready, share what you've been going through and ask for forgiveness. The relationships were damaged; approaching people to try to reconnect can't leave the relationship any worse off than it already is, so why not give it a shot?

If you don't feel you can face your addiction alone or want extra guidance, get professional help.

There is no shame in admitting you need help. You are taking on a difficult task. Any tools you feel would be useful are worth seeking out. Maybe you would benefit from seeing a psychologist who specializes in eating disorders or any issues you may be dealing with, like divorce, illness, loss of a loved one, loss of a job, disability, etc. They can help you find ways to cope with the stressors in your life, instead of reaching for food or doing other behaviors that may be hurting you. For me, that hour I go for counseling is a release; I get to say whatever I want, without fear of being judged or that someone in my life may find out my thoughts when I'd rather keep it to myself. Sometimes it is nice to get another person's perspective, especially if they are not directly involved in your life. Maybe you'd like to see a dietitian who specializes in disordered eating. If you don't feel that it is helping, you don't have to continue going. But don't give up after your first try. You may not click with the first person you choose to see. You should feel comfortable sharing with them. It may take time.

Some people are wired to feel like they don't need help. We all need help sometimes. I like to think of a counselor as a coach. If I need help training my body, I get a personal trainer. If I need help training my brain, I get a counselor. Don't be ashamed of getting help! Asking for help does not mean you are weak; it takes courage to admit that you need help getting through your struggles. Don't let anyone tell you differently.

Leaning on People Can be Difficult

When Chet and I moved back to the area where my family is from, I ended up wanting to help with the care of my Gram. She had a stroke during the time I lived in Virginia and my family decided to keep her home and care for her on their own. Keeping her out of a nursing home was my family's goal and I wanted to contribute as best I could. I would visit during the week and try to help with meals, her hygiene, or help get her to her appointments. I tried to help my uncle out on weekends too... he lived with her and spent evenings and weekends providing her care. He would never complain, but it was obviously stressful. I never felt like I did enough.

It was hard to see the woman I looked up to most deteriorate like she did…. she had been a strong, independent person. Over a few years' time she lost most of her mobility and ended up staying in her living room, where she slept in a hospital bed. You could tell it took a lot of effort to do simple things many of us take for granted, like walk to the commode, wash her face or brush her teeth. Helping her shower often overwhelmed me. I did my best to act like it was no big deal, but to have to bathe the woman who once cared for me... to have to help her with her lotion, get her dressed and do her hair, made me sad. It was also a physically exhausting task to help her in and out of the car, help her into her wheelchair and push her up the ramp to get inside. I tried to act like it was no big deal if none of the men were free to help... I was a strong girl. I could tell she felt like a burden. I never wanted her to feel that way... none of us did, but when you have to completely rely on others it can do bad things to your sense of worth. I'd paint on my happy face and try to lighten the mood with my goofy antics. I'd get her settled, hang out with my uncle, and try to pretend it didn't bother me. I didn't want to share with my family how hard it was for me because I didn't want to let anyone down... especially her. I barely liked to admit it bothered me... denial helped me get through it. But there were times I felt helpless... like I couldn't do enough for her. I couldn't take her struggles away, and that was all I ever wanted to do. Sometimes I would go home and binge on some of my favorites to "make me feel better". Then I'd get to feel like crap about me again, which was more familiar and I suppose, comforting in a way.

I recognized I used food to cope at this point, but the strong feelings I had about Gramma's situation were often too much for me to process. I had a lot of people who loved and supported me, but I still didn't know how to lean on them. Having that safety net is different from knowing how to use it. Also, I felt like I shouldn't be feeling the way that I did. It wasn't like I had it the worst of all of us... clearly Gram had the most difficulties, and my uncles, father and aunt, who provided the most care. The guilt I felt for feeling like it was hard to care for her often overrode what I had been learning about emotional eating, and I kept doing it. That's when I realized I should go for counseling again. I was a student at Marywood at the time. The months prior to her passing were especially hard and I broke down in class. One of my professors suggested I go to the student counseling center. I wasn't aware that they had free services for students, which is common at most colleges and universities. Having that hour to myself every week to vent felt freeing. It was hard to look at the truth behind how I felt, but acknowledging all those different, confusing feelings and getting validation for them helped me not reach for food.

God… The Ultimate Safety Net

God has been a big part of my safety net for many years. He is something I tend not to talk about. I guess I consider my relationship with Him private. I know from reading this book you wouldn't think I consider anything private, but at this point it is not something I'd like to say too much about. Although I have a little I'd like to convey…

I first started talking to Him in Virginia when I was at the lowest point I had been thus far in my life. I felt sick, broken, unseen, exhausted and at the end of my rope. I had been bouncing from doctor to doctor for a couple years and no one could tell me anything besides the fact that I needed to lose weight, which I kept failing at repeatedly. One night when I couldn't sleep I searched the internet again for something that may give me a clue as to what to do with myself. In that moment I felt completely lost and hopeless. I dropped to my knees in the middle of my bedroom and sobbed and asked God to help me. I told Him I couldn't do this anymore and I certainly couldn't do it without his strength and guidance. I sobbed for a while, but then suddenly got this sense of peace. Somehow, I knew He was listening and would start directing me.

I've talked to Him every day since that day. I often find comfort in knowing He is listening, guiding me if I'll listen. I often pray that He will light my path brightly because I can tend not to see it. For instance, I keep getting nervous because I'm not sure about how to get this book published. I'm not sure whether I should submit a proposal to a publishing company or self-publish. I feel like there is too much work left to be done and it gets overwhelming. Between thinking about editing, and all the other steps it is going to take to complete this project, it ends up terrifying me. The fear of the unknown strikes again! If I slow myself down and pay attention I can tap into what I'm supposed to be doing next, and I believe that's His guidance.

No matter what is going on, what concerns you have, God is always there to listen, to guide and to love and comfort you. I am certainly no spiritual advisor, but if building a closer relationship with Him is something that interests you I am sure there are people in your community who can help you do that. Don't give up. If you try a church that doesn't seem to fit, there are probably many more you can try right around the corner.

Chapter 12
What Happened After I Figured Out All This Stuff?

By Spring of 2007 I had been working on my emotional eating tendencies for almost four years. I learned how to tap into my feelings, process them and deal with them in healthy ways. When I looked at how I felt about my situation, I finally admitted I was miserable at work and it was time to make a change.

I enjoyed the staff I worked with at the hospital in the Admissions department, but I received a promotion to Supervisor with little supervisory experience. I was 26 at the time, one of the youngest on staff. I felt awkward telling folks what to do who were older and more experienced in the department, especially since I considered many of them my friends. I had little training. I got thrown into situations I wasn't prepared for, like firing, hiring and writing people up. I had gotten fed up with my job. I would buy lottery tickets on Sunday in hopes I would win and not have to go back there. I'd lose, and then spend the rest of the night crying or moping on my recliner.

At that time Chet was doing well at his job. He graduated the year prior and had been working as a broadcast engineer for about a year. We agreed that it was my turn to go back to school.

I had wanted to go back to school for nutrition since I figured out I was an emotional eater, which changed my whole view on life. I wanted to help patients and healthcare providers rewire their whole approach to weight loss and wellness, but I felt that I needed the credentials behind my name to add credibility. Who was going to listen to a chubby, formerly aspiring chemist when it came to weight loss? If I stayed at the 250-pound mark, one hundred pounds lighter than I had been previously, people still would consider me fat. I was afraid nobody would listen to me. I assumed they might be more likely to listen if I had the Registered Dietitian credentials after my name, and I might as well get the Master's degree while I was at it.

I was scared to go back to school. What the heck was I thinking?! I already had a Master's degree; was I going to commit to another 3-4 years of school? Could I really afford it? With a body mass index (BMI) of more than 35, I was considered morbidly obese. Was that allowed in a nutrition program? There were all these skinny girls in my classes who were at least ten years younger than me. Too fat AND too old?! What was I getting into?!

As it turned out I loved Marywood. I didn't end up feeling nearly as out of place as I imagined I would. I enjoyed all my classes. I loved Food Science. I made all the chemistry connections and I found it fascinating. I took the graduate level Biochemistry for Nutrition majors. I also took another graduate level course, Nutrition and Human Behavior. We talked a lot about emotional eating. I was encouraged to share my experience. It was refreshing to know that there were professors at Marywood who knew what I was talking about. I was intellectually stimulated for the first time in a long time. I felt alive. I knew I made the right decision. I was the happiest I had been in years, at least for that first week....

Then it All Started to Fall Apart

September of 2007 is when it all went downhill for Chet, which coincidently was my first week back at school. He was at work. It was late at night. His buddy was driving a pickup back to the TV studio from a remote site. A stretch of road that was being worked on wasn't clearly marked. His coworker didn't see that the road was stripped down quite a bit. When he pulled into the other lane the vehicle flipped several times. They were lucky to be alive.

The photos of the truck afterwards were shocking. It was totally wrecked.

I will never forget that night. I was at my Gram's house, talking with Uncle Mike. Gram was admitted to the hospital at the time. It was around 11:30 PM. I picked up the phone, assuming Chet was home safe, but instead he said "Julie, I love you." That's never how he started a conversation so I knew something was wrong. He explained what happened and he thought he was bleeding from his head. I told him I loved him but he better get off the phone and put pressure on his head until help got there. It took him 45 minutes to call me back. That was one of the scariest times of my life. It seemed to take an eternity.

Chet told me they got to the hospital and he was ok. His head throbbed and his eyes hurt, but he was going to be fine. He was extremely jumpy for weeks afterwards. He dreamed of the rollover a lot. He'd thrash in his sleep and say "NO, NO, NO!" He started seeing a counselor and psychiatrist for meds. He was put on Xanax and that helped take the edge off overnight. He couldn't take it during the day since it made him too sleepy. His shoulder ached for a while after the accident. His head hurt and his eyes were sensitive.

I recommended that he go to an eye doctor to follow-up. The doctor saw that his one eye seemed to have decreased blood-flow and sent him to a neurologist, who would be better qualified to handle the case. He said the eyes themselves were fine. Chet got an appointment with the neurologist and he did MRIs and MRAs of the head and neck. Gram was ill at the time and I didn't think about those test results. The day after she passed away we got a phone call from the doctor questioning Chet about stroke-like symptoms. He explained to him that his carotid was almost completely blocked and he needed to take aspirin, take it easy and see the vascular surgeon as soon as possible. He said that blocked carotids can occur from trauma; the vertebrae can nick the blood vessel, causing clotting around it and block it. It is called a dissection. The artery could also stretch out like a rubber band and not snap back like it should. It could be both narrower than it should be and blocked. We were both scared.

The vascular surgeon set him up for a cardiac cath the next week. He said that one of two things could happen. Either they could fix the carotid with a stent or, if necessary, they could do surgery the next day, an endarterectomy, to scrape out the blockage. Either way it sounded like it would be fixed, but it was scary.

Turns out that they couldn't do the stent or the surgery because the blockage went up into his brain. The doctor said it wasn't plaque, it was definitely scar tissue and clots. The blood flow to the brain was considered normal because the other arteries took up the slack. The vascular surgeon basically said to continue the aspirin and continue with his daily life. The whole thing didn't make sense. One minute they told the man he was going to have a stroke, and the next minute they told him to go about his usual business. Sure doc… no problem!!!

Chet had trouble with his workman's comp insurance covering his medical expenses. They said you couldn't prove the carotid blockage was from the accident and they wouldn't pay for any follow-up testing or second opinions. The doctors said it was from a trauma and this was the only trauma Chet encountered in his lifetime. How else would be have gotten it if not from the accident?! Gotta love insurance companies. Our regular medical health insurance wouldn't cover second opinions either, but at least someone covered all the initial testing and hospital stay.

Almost Dropped out of School

I enjoyed Marywood as much as I could given the circumstances. Not only had Chet's accident thrown us for a loop, but Gram's health had been declining. She was one of my best friends... my best cheerleader. Her home felt like my own. Anytime I needed comfort I knew I could turn to her. It was hard to watch her become progressively weaker. She passed away during the break after Christmas. Many of us got to be with her that day. It was an emotional time.

Between Gram's passing and Chet's health issues, I felt like I couldn't take much more stress. We buried Gram on January first, found out about Chet's carotid that next day, and I found myself back in school the following week, crying in class when the professor made reference to the fact that her break had been tough since her kids had gotten lice. Lice?! I burst into tears, thinking I wish freaking lice were the only thing I had to handle. She ended up letting the class take a break and talked with me for a minute. She hooked me up with the information I needed for Student Counseling and the Office of Retention in case I needed to take some time off.

I decided that it was too big of a risk that I took to go back to school and my goals were too important to be put on hold. I feared if I took time off that I wouldn't get to come back. I decided to go to counseling weekly and continue in the program. I continued exercising most days of the week to help keep my stress level down.

The Anxiety Continued

Chet's anxiety level had been high since his accident. Almost two and a half years passed and it got increasingly difficult for me to handle. Chet had a hard time driving after the accident. He was more cautious than normal and worried about me being on the road. He had outbursts too, talking about how he should have died in the accident. A commercial came on one night for OnStar and he started crying. He said he could still see it happening, that he was rolling and rolling and praying that God would keep him alive so he could see me again. He did more crying that two years after the accident than I saw him do in the previous fifteen. I tried to support him as best I could, but often there was little I could do to soothe him.

A year after the accident Chet found out he would probably be let go from his job due to cuts in the state budget. It had nothing to do with his work performance; he was one of the low men on the totem pole. He was well-liked; no one had anything bad to say about him. He loved that job and knowing he was going to lose it made his anxiety and depression get worse.

Chet was let go in August of 2009. He started getting more depressed. He'd lay on the couch all the time. He'd sleep in late. He wouldn't do much all day. He'd just sit and think about his "shitty life". I wouldn't care if he were sitting around relaxing, enjoying himself. He worked for 37 years straight… he deserved a break. Instead I felt he dug himself deeper into a hole. All I could do was watch him do it. Nothing I did or said seemed to help. He tried several medications. He'd been seeing a therapist and we started going for marriage counseling too. The severity of his depression and anxiety put a huge strain on our marriage. I was a full-time student in a graduate program and an internship program. I was teaching classes, too. It was challenging. I could barely deal with all this other stuff on top of it. My mood hadn't been the most stable.

I felt like the marriage counseling made Chet more aware of how his behaviors were affecting me. I thought that would be a good thing, but all it did was make him feel like he was no good for me. We started to work on drawing boundaries between us so that he could work on himself and I could work on myself. It's easy to get sucked into depression, especially if you have a tendency towards low moods. All it seemed to do was push him into a darker place. I spent most of my winter break wondering what the heck to do for him and with him.

Over the years I did all I could for Chet. I listened and tried to draw things out of him. I encouraged him to go for therapy. I went with him. I gave him many books to read and journals to write in. I prayed with and for him. I went to church with him. I included him in as many family and friend gatherings as I could. I encouraged him to make friends of his own and talk to as many people as he could. I gave him as much love and support as I had to give. I wrote him letters and sung him songs. I played music for him. I tried to take whatever negative thing he said and turn it around into a positive. I took him to the woods for walks as often as possible, since he felt more peaceful there. I hung up posters with positive sayings. I gave him supplements and tried to get him to eat better and exercise. I bought him a sunlamp for light therapy. I lit candles for him. I tried aromatherapy. I cheered him on for years. I exhausted myself. It got to the point when I didn't feel like I could do it anymore. I didn't know what to do. I was losing myself.

Backslides Happen
8.4.09

This summer I've reverted to some old ways. I have done well with not emotionally/mindlessly eating for over the last year and a half, but I feel like I completely overextended myself lately and have let myself go. I felt exhausted, mentally, and physically, after my internship hours were completed at the end of June. Suddenly, I completely changed my lifestyle. I stopped exercising. I stopped eating well. Hardly ate any fruits and veggies at all. Had 2-3 candy bars a day for three weeks. Three or four nights a week I had 8 cans of beer. All I wanted to do was sit on my recliner and watch TV. I watched more TV this month than I had in the past year.

I know it has been a rough couple of years since I started school, but I try not to focus on our problems so I can function. My friend Nikol said that it sucks that crap seems to hit the fan every time I'm in school. In VA we had lots of drama…. I got my Master's in Chemistry while I was exhausted, gained weight at rapid rates, had surgery for tumors on my ovaries, got diagnosed with depression, Chronic Fatigue Syndrome, Irritable Bowel Syndrome and PCOS. Chet was let down when the job he was promised didn't go through and he couldn't find a better one the whole time we were there. His depression got so bad that he started having suicidal thoughts and I had to hospitalize him. So much drama. Then when I started school this time around, Gram got sick the first week of school after we buried her beloved dog and Chet was in his rollover. By the time that January rolled around I thought that I would have to quit school. Gram passed away over winter break and the day after the funeral we got a call about Chet's carotid being blocked. They thought he may have a stroke. I cried every day for at least two months. Gram was one of my best friends. I missed her deeply, but had to worry about one of my other best friends, my husband. Then, another one of my best friends got his heart ripped out by his cheating wife. I worried for him and cried as I listened to his pain for months afterwards. So, I spent most of 2008 crying or being stressed out. On top of all that drama I had to concentrate on school. I also taught a biochemistry lecture for the first time that year. I managed to keep my 3.95 GPA, which should give an idea of how much time I spent on school as well. No wonder why I am so freaking tired.

Last time I had a stint of overeating and realized it as it was happening was when Gram died. It lasted a few weeks. I gained 10 pounds. I felt out of control. I felt so guilty. I felt like I should know better. I felt like since I was writing a book about binge eating, I should never do it again. I felt like I failed. It was only a few weeks.

This time it's been about a month. I feel differently about it. I feel like I'm so tired that I don't care. Not only do I not care, but I don't care that I don't care. And that thought does kinda scare me, but not enough to change my behavior. I also know I've gained weight, but I don't care. I figure this phase will pass soon and I'll drop the 10 or so pounds I gained and forget about it. I am forgiving myself while I am behaving in a way that I know is unhealthy and hypocritical. Interesting.

I know I have all these tools that I can use to help me feel better. I can vent to friends on the phone, write in my journal, talk to Chet, hike, read, sing, dance, listen to music. The list of things I like to do to blow off steam is very long. At the bottom of the list is still "eat" and "drink". Right now I don't want to do any of the other things on the list. I want to eat and drink. I wonder if there will be a day when these two words won't appear on my list anymore.

Shortly after this entry I snapped myself out of it. I started exercising regularly again, sleeping better and eating healthier foods. I quit binge drinking. I went for counseling again and wrote in my journal more. I forgave myself quickly. The road I started to go down was a scary one, but it was familiar. I knew how to pump the brakes and reroute myself. In the past I could have stayed in that funk for a long time and gained a lot of weight in the process. In extreme life circumstances we are more likely to fall back into old behaviors. But, if you keep working on new behaviors it will become easier to get back to taking better care of yourself. It gets easier to hit that reset button.

With more Practice, the Backslides Can Be Avoided
2.24.10

I am thankful that I've taken the path I've been traveling. If I hadn't uncovered my emotional eating many years ago, I'm sure I wouldn't have dealt with everything that's been going on as well as I have been. The thought of Chet wanting to be dead… hearing his counselor read his words out loud makes me incredibly sad for him. The thought of him not being here breaks my heart. Knowing that there is nothing I can do to get him to see the world in a positive light, that he doesn't get joy from anything anymore, and that there is no way of telling how long he is going to be like that…. it disturbs me immensely. I know how to deal with it though.

I haven't done any emotional eating during the last few months. I have pulled out the full arsenal of tools I built to deal with stress…. I've called friends, written in my journal, meditated, prayed, lit candles, sung songs, exercised, taken naps, gotten a massage, gone to the movies, gone shopping, and managed to work on stuff for school. I haven't had anything to drink either. I'm pleased that I can deal with the intense anxiety I've been feeling. I am allowing myself to feel my feelings and process them. I know they won't drag me down forever.

If you are not used to doing it, allowing yourself to feel your feelings can be overwhelming at times:

3.12.10

I spent years trying to uncover the feelings that were disguised as hunger. Now, with everything going on in my life, more specifically with my husband's depression, anxiety, PTSD, mixed bipolar disorder and recent suicidal thoughts, I have felt so many different things at once that it's hard for me to believe this is all inside me. Recently I've felt…

- Sad for Chet. Knowing that he wakes up every day wishing he were dead… knowing that he can't see the world through my eyes and see how truly beautiful life is absolutely breaks my heart.
- Frustrated. Chet is mixed up right now and there is nothing I can do for him except communicate as best I can with his healthcare team as to what I've observed. I'm frustrated with the whole situation… with the care he's gotten that hasn't been enough, with all the drugs they've had him try that haven't worked, with the way he approaches everything in a negative way, and hasn't been able to do all the things that everyone tells him to do.

- More frustrated. Frustrated with the people who can't seem to give me a break either, despite the fact that they know what's going on in my life… it's important to make up that snow day I guess, huh? Even if it means I have to miss an important meeting with one of Chet's doctors?
- Frightened. Way deep down in the bottom of my heart there is this fear that Chet has killed himself any time I haven't gotten him on the phone, especially when I know he should be available. I've been told by many people to keep the faith and trust that he will be ok. I've been told that it's in God's hands. If something does happen there is no way for me to stop it. I'm not in control. Is that supposed to make me feel better?! As different as Chet has been, I have to believe deep down that he is the man that I fell in love with. That man is supposed to be with me, at least until he's old and dies of natural causes, not until he chooses to end his own life. All my dreams for the future have him in them. I honestly don't know what I'd do if he wasn't with me anymore and part of all I see happening in the future.
- Confused. Mental health is confusing. On one hand I know that there are brain chemicals that are screwed up in his head. On the other hand, I know there are things he could be doing to take better care of himself that may help him to balance out. I'm confused at the anger I have because I don't know what or who to blame for it. Is it Chet's fault that he feels bad? Is it the fault of the imbalanced chemicals in his brain?

- Guilt. Is it my fault? Have I done things for or to him that have made his depression worse? Have I made him feel somehow that he isn't enough for me or that he's failed me?
- Sad for me. I miss my husband. The man I married was different from the man I live with now… most of the time I feel like he is a stranger.
- Disconnected. I don't feel like I can share everything with everyone that I consider important in my life. Mental illness is poorly understood and weirds out a lot of people. I don't want anyone treating me or Chet any differently. I don't want anyone to blame Chet for all the stress he's put on me either.
- Like a burden. I know I've leaned very hard on those people I have felt I can share with… I've had to… I have felt like I'm getting sucked into his darkness. I know all my friends want to support me, but this has been going on for so long that I fear I'm wearing them out… some more than others.
- Like a liar. Most of the lies I tell are to protect our secrets, but it's so much to juggle. The mask I wear most of the time is good, but I know many people can tell my smile isn't genuine.
- Loyal. Even though I feel disconnected to him lately, I think I've done a good job of keeping up my end of the marriage vows.
- Lonely. I don't feel like he can support me right now. I don't feel like he has been able to see me for a long time. He's not the partner I thought I'd always have.

- Proud. I've wanted to throw in the towel all semester and I haven't. I haven't wanted to go to school most days. I'm not enjoying it like I generally do, but at least I'm doing it…. even if it isn't my best effort.
- Angry. I've been extremely upset that all this is happening right now… what timing! I can't believe I had to commit my husband once and almost twice in one of the most difficult semesters in this program. I'm angry he hasn't worked harder over the years to build an arsenal of coping mechanisms to prevent falling into depression as deeply as he has, especially since he knows he has had tendencies towards depression. I'm angry I've had to do any of this… I can't believe I had to listen to him beg me to take him home from the hospital in the middle of the night, spend hours talking with the people that are supposed to be taking care of him, threatening him that he'd better get his shit together and make it his job to reprogram his thinking because I honestly don't know how much longer I can take it, go to all these appointments, go to therapy for myself, etc., etc.… all this time taken up when I could be enjoying the fact that I personally feel better than I have felt in years… that I finally will get to do the very thing I feel I was meant to do. And I feel so selfish about that thought.
- Unstoppable. I know that no matter what happens in my personal life I will spread the message I was meant to spread.
- Overwhelmed. So many days to get logged in for the supervised practice for my internship. So

```
much to log and report. So many little
projects. So many quizzes and tests. So many
lab reports to grade. So much research I have
to do for my thesis. So many doctor's
appointments to attend. So many thoughts to
organize in my head. So much time I would need
to process all that's going on… time that I
don't have.
```
• **Exhausted. Who wouldn't be?**

Divorce

We had not given each other what we needed for years and I finally allowed myself to accept my conclusion that we were doing more harm than good by staying together. It was a toxic situation; I was losing myself for years and was starting not to recognize myself. Right after Christmas of 2010 we had our last argument in the house. I sat on the couch sobbing. He barely looked at me. I knew it was over. I packed up a bag and left.

I drove up to Scranton and stayed the night at my sister's. The next day I went down the street to my parents and asked to move in with them. They were shocked. My family knew that Chet was depressed, but they didn't know the extent of it, or what it was doing to me and our marriage. Again, I had wanted to protect Chet so I didn't share the details of his struggles. I also didn't want them to blame him for putting stress on me.

As I sat in a pile of tissues, curled up on the bed in the room I grew up in, crying uncontrollably, I realized that had my marriage ended any time earlier than it did, I would not have been able to deal with it. If I had eaten myself through the pain, I would have gained hundreds of pounds… and there was a time I literally could have. The sea of tissues would have been a sea of peanut butter cup wrappers and potato chip bags.

For a while I held onto the idea that maybe Chet and I could get back together. I thought I might have time to get back to being ok myself, then I'd try to help him again. I thought that my leaving might jump-start something in his brain and he'd work on things a little harder to fight for himself and for us. It wasn't working out that way.

4.12.11

I can't believe it's the middle of April. It's been 3.5 months since I moved out of the house. It all seems surreal. I've been trying my best to focus on the positive things in my life… I've been productive at times, writing my thesis and writing articles for Livestrong, running, talking with friends, praying and journaling… but at night before bed when it's me and my thoughts I get so sad.

Sad isn't a good enough word for it. It has felt like I'm broken… like my heart and soul have been ripped in half. I invested valuable time in us… I never expected something that I worked so hard for would turn out so bad.

I miss… coming home to him, talking about my day with him and listening about his, eating dinner together, watching movies and cuddling on the couch, playing Scrabble, going for walks/hikes together, having picnics, sleeping with him…

And it may not seem like much, but if you think about it our days are filled with all those day-to-day interactions. I thought I found someone I liked being around all the time and I could settle for that. But I needed more and I didn't get it for a long time. I couldn't give him what he needed either.

There are many triggers for my sadness. I was sad when I saw the cherry blossoms on the trees... we had such a good time going to the festival in DC. Remembering those good times makes me long for more of them. I was sad when I saw his favorite chocolate cake, Oreo cookies, marshmallow bunnies, daffodils (he planted them for me), pictures of us together, etc. I get sad when I think about all the things he was supposed to be involved in... supposed to share with me... my birthday, Easter, every other holiday to come, my thesis defense, graduation, my first book launch/signing, my first job as a dietitian...

And while I may miss all these things or I am sad for what we won't share together, now if I think about it and allow myself to feel it, I know that our marriage is broken beyond repair.

Filing

November of 2011 I filed for divorce. It was official in April of 2012. It was one of the hardest things I've ever had to do. I care for him deeply despite all that happened between us. I knew him for half of my life. I pictured us being friends after the divorce, but that hasn't been the case. I pray for him. I know he still struggles. Thinking about it breaks my heart. Many people suffer with depression in silence. It is my hope that more people start to share their struggles and get the help they need. There is no shame in admitting you need help. It takes a strong person to reach out.

Getting Divorced AND Looking for a Job?!

While trying to find a job, I lived with my parents for six months after I left my husband. Talk about stress. I never thought I'd find myself living at home again, completely leaning on my family for financial support while trying to process that I left the man I promised to be with until "death do us part". I felt like a complete failure... yet again. It was probably good that I had the time off to sit in my emotional wreckage, but it sure didn't feel good at the time. I was fortunate that my friends and family helped see me through it.

I was hired at a major medical center in Danville, PA in June of 2011. I moved there the following month. It was an amazing feeling to be out on my own again, collecting a paycheck and doing work as a dietitian. I had a job where I knew I'd be able to spread awareness of emotional eating, yet I wasn't enjoying it. I spent months being stressed out, often stayed late to finish my work, and found myself crying quite a bit. Starting my life over from scratch was proving to be quite difficult.

I decided to give a talk for my new peers on my experience with emotional eating. I wanted them to understand my history, and hopefully shed light on where many of their patients were coming from. My message was better received than I imagined it would be. I started making friends within the department and I felt comfortable there. My office became like a second home. I've gotten a lot of love and support from the staff over the last few years.

After filing for divorce, having the stress of having a second job as a dietitian in a local community hospital, and having my divorce get finalized, I was quite sad. One of my new friends, who will be called HC from this point forward, looked at me one day and said, "You've been sad for a long time." She pointed out the obvious, but moving forward I decided to work on snapping myself out of it. I often talk about how people need to be their own best cheerleaders and get off the couch to get more physically active. One of my new favorite analogies is that people need to get off their "emotional couch". We often spend too much time thinking about the past and mourning the idea of how we thought our lives would turn out. There comes a time when you need to snap yourself out of it. One of the most important things I did was to stop making "anniversaries for sad things" (HC's advice), like feeling bad when the one-year mark passed from when I decided to leave my husband. Or how when every holiday passed I'd think about how it was the first time Chet wasn't there for it. I needed to stop picking at that scab and keeping that wound open.

Chapter 13
PMS, Depression, and Anxiety

By this point in your reading you can tell that I've had a lot of depression, anxiety and PMS to fight. It has affected me my whole life, but I didn't realize how severe it was until this past year. It was my "norm".

I believe my most important gift is that I can share "embarrassing" or taboo things that most people wouldn't talk about freely. This hasn't always been the case. Unfortunately, in our society there is a stigma attached to mental health issues, even for common things like anxiety and depression. Depression has affected many people in my life, including myself, yet it hasn't been talked about too much. I have been trying to fight this tendency with many of my loved ones. Keeping it in and not sharing leads to feeling isolated, which often makes it worse.

I had first been depressed in middle school, mostly due to feeling bad about not being able to protect my friend from being molested, and about being overweight. It took a strong hold of me in high school. I cannot say I was suicidal; I wasn't close to doing it, but I wished I were dead for a while. I didn't tell anyone at the time. Maybe if I reached out it wouldn't have affected me for so long. It wasn't until I started running and joined the cross-country team my senior year that I started to feel better. I'm sure it was a combination of the endorphins, the weight loss, and especially the camaraderie. I felt stronger, more confident... happier in general. I made new friends and got a lot of support and encouragement from that group, as well as from the coaches.

Depression can manifest itself in different ways. For me, depression felt like a heaviness. I felt like gravity was stronger for me… like I was literally tied down. It was extremely difficult to get out of bed. I didn't give a shit about anything. I didn't care if I went to school. Didn't care if I did my homework. Didn't feel like hanging out with people, although I managed to do that anyway – I think it was part of the mask I wore.

I dug myself out of that depression in high school, but I had tendencies towards low moods and anxiety. This has always been the case, especially during PMS times. The sadness got worse when I got mono my senior year of college and had to stop running. I ended up gaining weight, being tired all the time, and becoming more depressed. I had issues with my memory and had to take time off from my schooling. I would forget to do many day-to-day things, like pay the bills or do laundry… oh yeah, or shower or wash my hair. That's why many of my "before" pictures show me with a handkerchief on my head. Every task seemed like it would take an enormous amount of energy, and simple things appeared overwhelming.

For years I was fake because I didn't know how to be real. I felt like I had to wear the mask of a happy person so I could fit in. I couldn't be fat AND wear a puss face…who would want to hang out with that girl? I was used to being everyone's clown. I felt like since I was good at being goofy, making people laugh and feel better, that somehow that was my duty.

For years I was fake because I thought I had to be to survive. Not only did I put my happy face on for my loved ones, but I did it for myself too. If I admitted how awful I felt at times, I would have had to deal with it. Pretending to be ok is how I coped with life. Ironically, the most difficult time I had putting up that façade was when I supported my ex-husband when he was suicidal. I hid his depression because I thought I had to; I didn't want anyone to look at him differently or feel like he was a burden. I hid his depression as well as my own. I felt like if I acknowledged how difficult it was I wouldn't have been able to do what I was doing… I would have fallen apart and not been able to continue with my schooling. I was a full-time student at the time when he was at his worst. I was an undergrad student, a graduate student, a dietetic intern, and part-time faculty at the school. I didn't think I could juggle all those balls if I admitted how I felt.

I can finally be real. Now I realize that I don't have to put on a show for my loved ones. I have to pull it together to see my patients and do my job, but I don't have to put on a front for the people that care about me. I first started to realize this when I fell into a darkness when I left my husband. When I finally admitted that I couldn't do it anymore, it was like my whole view on life changed. For years all I knew was supporting him. He was suicidal for a long time, and fights his depression to this day. For years we both went for counseling… he went separately, I went separately, we went together. We prayed together, went to church, listened to preachers, meditated, exercised, and he tried many different combinations of medications. We did everything we could. I became more of a caregiver than a wife; he was more of a patient than a husband. It was killing my spirit. I was losing myself.

When I finally left my husband I spent weeks crying non-stop, which tapered off to several hours a day after a couple months. I had headaches and couldn't sleep. I didn't want to eat. If I did, I only wanted Ramen noodles or peanut butter cups. I think I lived on those for a couple months. And yes, I did have a more difficult time distinguishing between my emotional hunger and need for comfort, versus actual, physical hunger at times. However, I didn't gain much weight… maybe a few pounds over about six months. I find that quite remarkable, because had I not put all these coping mechanisms into place that I outlined in this book… had I not journaled, talked with friends, gone for counseling, meditated, prayed, exercised, sang songs, etc.... I'm sure I could have eaten myself up to four or five hundred pounds in time.

My nervous energy also helped me maintain my weight during that time. This was a different way that my anxiety manifested itself from what I experienced in the past. I couldn't sit still for very long. It took six months to find a job after I left my husband. In my "free" time I started running a lot more. I also walked all over Scranton. I remember walking for several hours in the rain one day with my Dad's giant umbrella, while crying off and on. I cleaned all the time. I felt overwhelmed with any clutter around. I started to clean out closets, cupboards, attic spaces... you name it, I cleaned it. The movement helped me feel ok. I know it helped me sleep. It certainly helped me keep my weight steady.

Our Brain Chemicals

The brain is awesome. Not like totally cool awesome, though it is... awesome, as in causing awe. It commands our entire body. It is what makes us unique. There are different parts of the brain that do different things; however, all brain cells communicate in the same way. The neurons, brain cells, have gaps between them called synapse. Electrical impulses are fired off between them that can cause the release of different chemical messengers that will then bind with the next neuron. Those messengers are called neurotransmitters (brain hormones). The process repeats itself until the message has been relayed to different body parts, processed, and carried out. Just like other hormones, it reminds me of when we would pass notes in class in school.... think of each student as a brain cell, and the notes are the chemical messengers.

Neurotransmitters, as well as other hormones in our body, are often likened to a key. The receptor sites, where the neurotransmitters interact on the neurons, and other cells in the body, are often likened to a lock. The correct messages are sent when the right number of keys are opening the right amount of locks. This type of communication can break down and malfunction if the neurotransmitters are not balanced, like the symphony analogy I mentioned in the PCOS chapter.

There are receptor sites on the brain for the sex hormones, estrogen, progesterone, and testosterone. These are some of the main players in PCOS and they are often imbalanced. If they are not present in the proper amounts, it is understandable how PMS, depression, anxiety and other mood disorders can arise. It is not only our imagination and it doesn't make us weak. It means we need to rebalance ourselves.

There are many chemicals that impact our brain. The main ones that you've probably heard of that influence our mood are serotonin, dopamine, and norepinephrine (noradrenaline). These chemicals are made from amino acids, the building blocks of protein, in the presence of vitamins and minerals, to help the enzymes work correctly. This is one of the reasons it's so important to eat a variety of fruits and veggies… to get those vitamins and minerals in your system.

The most well-known brain chemical is serotonin. The antidepressants in the category of selective serotonin reuptake inhibitors (SSRIs), such as Zoloft, Prozac, Celexa and Lexapro are popular for treating depression and anxiety. As many people have pointed out, a Zoloft or Prozac deficiency does not cause depression. These drugs can temporarily control the symptoms of depression, but they do not fix the underlying problems. This is especially the case if you have situational depression, a low mood caused by a specific event in your life, such as an illness or loss of a loved one. Counseling is often a big help. I believe we can have better brain chemistry if our entire body is working more efficiently. If we give it the proper fuel, vitamins and minerals, sleep, exercise, sunlight, and treat ourselves with the same kindness and forgiveness that we give others, all those healthy behaviors can help us balance our brain chemicals.

Neuroplasticity is a new science that studies how the messages we send ourselves, the thoughts we have, change the signals being sent in our brain. You can purposely plant seeds of positivity in your brain to help them grow. There is something to this positive thinking stuff... it literally can change your brain for the better!

I am not telling you to take medications or not to take medications. Everyone's situation is different. While I had all my other physical problems, I also had depression, anxiety and mood swings. I cried every day, several times a day depending on the circumstances. I felt like everything was coming down on top of me. While attending UVA, I got to the point where I couldn't go anywhere without crying in public, including school, my workplace at the time. I would not be able to do anything about the rest of my health until I got my depression under control. I took Celexa for almost a year. I figured if I sprained my ankle, I would use an elastic support until it healed. Why wouldn't I do the same with my brain? Celexa would be the elastic. Once I got the proper dose, I no longer melted down in public. It helped me to be more productive.

When I took the Celexa I felt weak, as is common with depression. I felt like a loser because I couldn't handle what life dealt me. Isolating myself made the whole experience worse. I didn't talk about how I felt because I didn't think anyone could help. I know now that I was wrong. You can feel better by getting things off your chest. You can feel better having someone empathize with you and validate your feelings. Knowing people love you and support you can go a long way. I was lucky I could have talked with friends and family, but I didn't know how to talk. Now I try to share how I feel when I feel it, not three years later. I often thought about joining internet support groups, but I never did. I think they are valuable depending on your situation. It is comforting to know that people know what you are going through and won't judge you.

As I mentioned before there are receptor sites for progesterone, estrogen, and testosterone throughout our whole body, including our brain. There are more estrogen receptors in the cortex and limbic regions than in other areas of our brain. The limbic system is the major center for regulating mood, memory, sleep, sex drive, appetite, and pain. The fluctuation of estrogen alters serotonin, which then produces changes in all areas of our life. Changes in hormone levels, like those during menstrual cycles, puberty, pregnancy, and menopause will affect the amount of neurotransmitters made, as well as the sensitivity of the receptor sites towards the neurotransmitters. No wonder many women experience uncontrollable mood swings, depression, anxiety, PMS, memory loss, concentration difficulty, food cravings, fatigue, and insomnia, among other issues throughout their lives. Women do not merely fabricate these symptoms. They are real symptoms with real causes.

A whole host of symptoms can be caused by fluctuating sex hormones. An interesting example was given in <u>Screaming to Be Heard: Hormone Connections Women Suspect ...and Doctors Still Ignore</u> (Vliet, 2000). Some women experience heart palpations and anxiety attack symptoms during premenopause, during the PMS time of their menstrual cycle or in menopause. Estrogen levels decrease in the ovaries, causing decreased estrogen in the brain, causing decreased brain endorphins, causing a burst of brain adrenaline (NE), causing brain-body response to the stimulation from the NE, causing an increase in heart rate, palpitations, rise in blood pressure, awakening from sleep, dilation of body blood vessels triggering hot flashes, sweating, butterflies in the stomach, diarrhea, and headaches. All from a decrease in ovarian estrogen!

And that is only one example. Endocrinology, the study of hormones, is fascinating. If you feel you have a hormonal imbalance, talk to your doctor about having them tested.

I spent years with imbalanced hormones. This lead to severe PMS, but I recently got some relief:

6.28.17

I wasn't going to add any more journal entries to my book at this point, but I couldn't help but share my PMS story. My moods have always been so low for about four to five days before my period would come. When I was younger, the hard part was that I never knew how long my cycle would be, so I never got to predict when that dark time would come. It's not like I assumed that I would feel horrible, but every month I'd end up feeling like the sidewalk fell from under my feet, regardless of what I did to stop it. I'd feel ugly. I'd lose my confidence. I'd cry uncontrollably. Even this book, something I believe in more than anything, was doomed fail during those days. I'd feel like I spent my life working on something that wasn't going to help people anyway… like I wasted my time. The other days during the month I'm happy, strong, and confident. It was a lot for my loved ones to absorb, but I just always thought that's how it had to be… that's all I knew.

I finally couldn't take it anymore. There are other life circumstances lately that have been stressful, and the PMS on top of it was too much to bear. A couple of years back, my gyn told me about taking an antidepressant a week or two before my period to help. Since you are only on it part-time and you often only need a low dose, women experience less side effects. I decided to try to keep fighting it on my own, but it wasn't working. No matter what I did, that ground would fall from under me and I'd go dark. I called her to ask about the Prozac last month.

Normally antidepressants are meant to keep your serotonin levels up. However, when you take Prozac cyclically for PMS, it works differently. It affects a chemical in your brain called ALLO (allopregnanolone), which is a breakdown product of progesterone. Progesterone falls every month as a normal part of a menstrual cycle right before your period comes. This drop makes the ALLO go down too, contributing to the PMS symptoms. Prozac would help the effect of this drop in ALLO feel less drastic.

I tried it last month, and it felt like a miracle! I wasn't ugly. The sidewalk didn't fall from under me. I kept my confidence. I could breathe easier. I didn't cry. I could sleep. It was awesome! I have felt like "me" now for a whole 7 weeks in a row for the very first time in my life. It's amazing! I'm hopeful it will continue to be the case. I had gone online to see if there were message boards about this, and lots of women report similar results. I'm so glad I tried it.

Fight the Darkness

PMS, depression and anxiety are liars. Don't listen to them. They tell you that you can't do certain things… like get off the couch, shower, or go out in public. They are lies. Don't believe them. Fight the lies with all you have and soon it will get easier. And please talk to people about it!!!

Regardless of the source of your darkness, you can choose to fight it. Yes, sometimes it is normal to be in a low mood. However, if it lasts longer than you think it should, or it is preventing you from living your life, it is time to start fighting it. Purposely change your focus. Purposely see what is good in your life. Fight to take better care of yourself, one step at a time.

10.24.13
I have spent a lot of my life hoping my future would be better. I've been missing my present.

Chapter 14
Expanding the Palate:
Wait, you mean I can Love Food?!

Last Summer (2012) I gave myself a break. I started focusing on me. I felt selfish. I worked on getting what I needed. I knew it was the only way to get rid of the funk I had been in. I focused on exercise. I became stronger every day. I felt empowered. Was I the same woman who at one point couldn't manage to get off the couch? Was I the same person for whom it took all the energy she had to get up to shower? I felt strong again and independent for the first time. I had confidence. Amazing things were happening. I started to forgive myself for leaving my husband. I also learned how to enjoy food. It was a whole new experience that I never imagined possible. It was an important piece of the puzzle in my recovery that had been missing for far too long.

You Can Love Food?

HC often invited me to her place for dinner and she is an amazing cook. I spent many evenings sitting across from her in her kitchen watching her cook. I soaked up whatever she said and did like a sponge. It was like attending my own personal cooking show on a regular basis. She uses as many fresh ingredients as possible. Fresh ingredients make dishes that taste more flavorful than processed foods. I started cooking too and trying new recipes, bouncing ideas off HC and sharing my creations with others. It opened a whole new world for me.

My body changed a lot during this time as well. I did not purposely set out to try to lose weight. However, I did weigh myself periodically, and since I moved to Danville I lost about another fifty pounds. It is a strange adjustment. For example, I'm often surprised at what size clothing I need to purchase… do I only need a large? One day in a fellow dietitian's office there were two different sized chairs. I sat in the larger one, thinking that my toosh wasn't going to fit into the smaller one. When I looked down I saw about one foot of room in the chair. Then when she got up to leave the room, I decided to see how well I fit into the other chair. Turns out I had inches of room on either side of me. It's strange when your brain can't keep up with the changes your body has made. I think part of the problem is that you don't get to see yourself that often, unless you spend a lot of time in front of a mirror. Sometimes when I do look in a full-length mirror, or get a glimpse of myself in a window while I'm running down the street, I'm surprised at my appearance. Since when can I fit into roller-coaster seats? Since when can I run six miles in the morning and have the energy to dance for hours at night? I'm sure I'll catch on.

For years food was my enemy. Food ruined my life. I hated it. It made me get fat. It made me hate myself. Because of food, I was ugly, lazy and stupid…. virtually unlovable. Food was the object of my addiction, the main coping mechanism I used to deal with life. I abused food, it didn't abuse me. It wasn't food's fault.

I used the same foods over the years to soothe myself. How many cups of Ramen noodles, bags of sour cream and onion chips, peanut butter cups, cookies, donuts, and macaroni and cheese can a girl eat and still enjoy? I'd stick to the same entrees too. I got into a pattern of eating the same things, whether I cooked at home or went out to eat. I found comfort in the familiarity of it all, but over time it got boring.

For a while I was happy, I learned to do other things to relieve stress and stopped obsessing about food. I didn't count calories, grams of fat, carbs, protein, etc. I didn't study the food labels of every single thing I put into my mouth, only to feel guilty about eating it. I got the physical hunger thing down, and practiced stopping when I was physically full. However, it took quite some time for me to realize that I could enjoy food. That food can and is allowed to satisfy me.

Many of the books I read talked about eating until "satisfied", but I never thought much about what that meant. A food can satisfy a craving. It can be a wonderful taste and/or texture in your mouth and leave you satisfied, even pleased, without being physically full. For example, I love rich desserts like cheesecake. Before I learned to stop when I was full, I could have eaten several slices in one sitting. Now I know that I can stop eating when I've had enough of that experience in my mouth. That's the moment that I'm satisfied. Now if I'd like cheesecake, I can literally be satisfied with one bite of it. I allow it to melt in my mouth, squish between my tongue and the roof of my mouth, and experience the wonderful sweet creaminess. I frequently skip dessert all together if I am full. I know I won't enjoy it as much if I'm not hungry, so I don't bother. I know to some this may seem completely crazy, but I assure you that the more you practice, this type of experience can happen for you too!

Satisfaction is different than being full. The word satisfaction itself implies enjoyment. ***We are allowed to enjoy our food.*** We deserve to experience pleasure in life, and that includes the pleasure and satisfaction that can occur from experiencing food. We are allowed to be content and happy after experiencing food. We don't have to beat ourselves up for consuming "x" amount of calories, fat, carbs, etc. We can be pleased, content, and move on with our day.

There are many different flavor combinations to try… foods that could make my mouth happy. *'Wait a minute… is she trying to say that food should be allowed to elicit an emotional response in me? I thought we were supposed to cut all emotional connections to food?!'* Right… that's what I thought for a long time, but we are allowed to and deserve to take pleasure in food. Our taste buds are a gift and we are allowed to enjoy this sense. It's taken time for me, but now…

6.9.13

Yesterday I felt that I reached a whole new level with food, going someplace I never thought I'd be able to go. I believe I experienced what a friend of mine may have referred to as a "foodgasm". I had been out to dinner with friends at the beach. I decided that I would purposely try things I've never tried before. I had it in my mind that scallops were often rubbery and tasteless, so I hadn't ordered them out in years. I also thought that maybe the only time I liked them was when they were wrapped in bacon (what doesn't taste great wrapped in bacon, right?!). The two diver scallops arrived on a bed of greens, whose name I can't remember, but the presentation was very attractive. They were perfectly cooked, lightly browned on the outside and wonderfully tender and smooth in texture on the inside. They were seasoned perfectly. It was a flavor explosion in my mouth. Then I chose lamb lasagna as my entrée. I only tasted lamb once before in a stew. It was amazing. It wasn't a red sauce, nor did it contain cheese. It changed my idea of what lasagna had to be. It had English peas and spinach in between the layers of perfectly cooked noodles. The sauce was a brown sauce that was very eye-appealing – opaque yet glossy looking. It was a rich dish and I enjoyed every bite. I thought for sure that would be the end to my complete contentment with food for the evening, but then I

was served my dessert, brie cheesecake with a
raspberry sauce drizzle. It was absolutely
delightful. The sharpness of the brie was perfect
against the sweetness. For a few bites I sat there
and closed my eyes, taking in the whole
experience. I shared it with the table and didn't
feel the need to eat it all myself or save it for
later. I didn't feel any guilt about the
experience; I only felt pleasure and satisfaction.
I finally understand that food is not my enemy. I
think I'm in love.

We are allowed to enjoy the taste of our food. We can also enjoy the meal planning, recipe seeking, shopping for the ingredients, meal preparation, and presenting it either to ourselves or to loved ones. It's like foreplay… the buildup to the big moment. It took a lot of practice, but I've allowed myself to fall in love with the whole process. Also, we can go out to eat and try new dishes, cuisines, and flavor combinations. I spent decades feeling guilty for everything I ate, so all of this seemed like such a foreign concept.

I enjoy going to restaurants and trying new things. Then I like to go home and try to do it myself. It's amazing what we can create right out of our own kitchens. If you can read and follow directions, you can cook. It does take a lot of energy/planning, but it is worth it. Food made from fresh ingredients tastes better than anything processed, and it usually tastes better than food you can order out, especially from chain restaurants.

If you, like me, hadn't done much cooking, this whole idea can seem overwhelming. If you eat out most days during the week, it's not like you will switch gears completely and start cooking most days of the week. Like any change in behavior that will stick, the more slowly you ease into it, the better. Start by choosing one recipe, buying the ingredients, and making that one meal. If you enjoy it, which I know you will, you can choose one day out of the week that will be convenient for you to cook. I like to cook on Sundays. I usually have the day off from work so I can take a chunk of time to prepare any meal I'd like.

I lived alone and often felt that it wasn't worth the effort to cook for myself. I started to invite friends or family to eat with me, which is always fun. However, sometimes that isn't possible. I decided if it were for me alone, I could and should cook myself exactly what I wanted. There are often leftovers, which you get to eat during the week or can freeze for later. You can also pass out leftovers to friends. They will appreciate it! You may find that your friends will do the same in return. It is fun to try other people's cooking, share recipes, and get new ideas.

People often use the excuse that it is too expensive to cook certain meals. New ingredients, such as herbs and spices can add to your grocery bill. However, if you make the commitment to cook, you will be getting your money's worth out of the new ingredients. I have friends who enjoy cooking from whom I've gotten herbs and spices if I only needed a small amount. I have also borrowed their kitchen gadgets. For example, I never used a food processor before and didn't have the cash to get one, so a friend let me borrow hers. I've borrowed all types of things. When I realize that I'm using the kitchen item more frequently than I thought I would, I purchase one for myself. Like a microplane for example… who the heck woulda thought I'd be zesting lemons?! Also, there are many stores that run good deals on kitchen supplies. If you take the time to shop around, you can probably find what you'd like to purchase at a fraction of the cost you thought you might have to spend.

You can feed at least 8 people with a lasagna that costs about $25 to make. That's only about $3 per person! What restaurant can you say that about? I'd much rather take the time to prepare the lasagna and only spend the $3 per serving than go for fast food and get a burger. People often complain about the cost of produce, but you can watch for sales and purchase the fruits and vegetables. You can go to your local farmers' markets or roadside stands to get cheap produce in season. If you truly can't afford fresh fruits and vegetables, the frozen products are lower in cost and often taste close to fresh.

The internet is a great source for recipes. I've often found it helpful to read people's comments that are attached to a recipe. The comments have often swayed me to use different spices, different amounts of ingredients, or add or subtract ingredients and they turn out great. It's nice to learn from others as we go. If you don't have access to the internet, you can find recipes not only in cookbooks, but also in the newspaper or magazines. Grocery stores often have handouts for meal suggestions.

After cooking this year, I've found myself being able to think about the ingredients I have on hand and put a meal together. HC often does that. Tonight, for example, she purchased butternut squash ravioli. I would have put store-bought sauce on them and called it a night. I knew that wasn't her plan. She had a variety of tomatoes on hand that she didn't want to go bad, so she roasted them in the oven. Then she added some wine to deglaze the roasting pan, added frozen peas, bacon, cream, and salt and pepper and put it back in the oven for a while. It all blended together into this wonderful, sweet and savory concoction to top the ravioli. Who wants store-bought sauce when you can whip this up at home?!

One of the first things I made at home that was out of my comfort zone was roasted veggies. They are easy to put together, delicious, and versatile. Roasting brings out full, bold, sweet flavor and you can roast any veggies you like. A friend had done zucchini, yellow squash, eggplant, onion, and cherry tomatoes and topped them with olive oil, balsamic vinegar, garlic and salt and pepper.

The roasting time varies depending on what veggies you do and what size pieces you cut. They do shrink as they roast. Learn from my mistake and make the pieces twice as big as you'll like them to be when they are done roasting. If you do too many at once, the veggies end up steaming themselves due to all the water that gets released, so make sure to spread one thin layer in the roasting pan or cookie sheet. They are done when they are nice and soft and some have golden brown edges. You can use the veggies any way you like… as a side dish to any meal, topping pasta, on a sandwich, or on a salad. Root veggies turn sweet in the oven. A mixture of carrots, parsnips, and sweet potatoes is yummy. Drizzle with a little olive oil and salt and roast away! It could take up to an hour. You can roast while doing other things in your home you'd like to get done, like paying bills, doing laundry, etc. It's nice to get other chores done and come back to a wonderful meal or snack that's been roasting for you.

My idea of what a salad can be has expanded this year. There are many different choices for greens for the base. You can add roasted veggies to the salad as well. One of my favorites from last year was a roasted beet salad that HC put together. She used dark greens, including spinach, roasted beets, goat cheese and sweet toffee-roasted almonds with a balsamic vinaigrette. So yummy, I could go for some right now! It's not like it is too hard to put together, but they are flavors I would not have thought to combine before. If you are intimidated by the idea of cooking, salads can be a great place to start. Preparing the salads can get you into the kitchen and using fresh ingredients.

You can expand your idea of the different foods you already know you enjoy. For example, I like toast or an English muffin with strawberry jelly. There are many combinations of different types of breads and jams and jellies to try. Fig jam is one of my new favorites. I didn't know it existed. I never looked before. Many grocery stores carry a great variety of foods. Do yourself a favor and peruse the aisles once in a while to check out all the new products that are becoming available.

Recipe modification… sometimes necessary, sometimes not. Chronic dieters everywhere gasped! Hahaha!!! Seriously though, we often get stuck on modifying ingredients… on substituting low-fat or fat-free for full-fat versions of foods or replacing white flour carbs with whole grains, that we miss out on many great flavors and consistencies. Yes, there are foods I will eat the low-fat versions of on a regular basis. Yogurt for example… most of the time I'm satisfied with the fat-free Greek, but I won't feel guilty if I prefer to eat the 2% fat yogurt if the flavor I would enjoy at that moment happens to be the higher-fat counterpart. Fat-free cheese is often tasteless. Reduced fat cheese is more satisfying. However, I would prefer to eat smaller quantities of the high-fat cheeses and enjoy the flavor. There are wonderful cheeses out there to introduce to your palate. Some can be quite expensive, but you'll be satisfied with a small amount. In general, you can be satisfied with a smaller quantity than you think you can.

I used to be hooked on sweet treats and I didn't often pay attention to appetizers, entrees, or side dishes. Many foods taste amazing in the savory real-food world. 'Savory real-food world… what the heck is that?!' you ask? That's what I call real foods made from whole, fresh ingredients after hanging out with HC. I'd rather have roasted veggies with balsamic and fresh basil than dessert most of the time. That's something I never thought I'd say!

10.20.13 Braciole night.

Food is love?! Oh man, it took me years to feel that wasn't the case. Was I wrong? It took two hours to look up recipes, compile a grocery list, and go to the store. It took another three hours to prepare the stuffed beef and homemade sauce. It took another hour to clean up. All that time and effort… obviously you don't go through all this work for people you don't love. So… food is love! For years I wanted to detach all emotion from food, but that's ridiculous. Sharing a delicious homemade meal at a nicely set dining room table with good company and great ambiance, good music, candles lit, etc… what's better than that?!

Respect

I have been thinking about respect lately. Respect… esteem for or a sense of worth… to hold in high regard. Many of us do not respect food. I know I didn't until recently. I feel that lack of respect stems from not considering all that goes into putting our food in front of us. Since many of us do not take the time to prepare our own meals, culinary skills and presentation are often taken for granted. We don't often think about the hard work it took to grow, harvest, and prepare the ingredients. We rush through our meals without truly tasting or appreciating them.

HC probably has the highest regard for food of anyone I've met thus far. She is always looking for new recipes or ingredients to try. I've seen all the work she puts into it and the outcome is worth the effort. I have a greater appreciation for food after watching her go through the entire process: finding the recipe, purchasing the ingredients, prepping, cleaning veggies and herbs, chopping, preparing meats, cooking, cleaning, serving, presenting and my favorite step… tasting, savoring and enjoying food. All of this takes a lot of time. I think if we cooked more often we'd be more likely to slow down and relish in the experience of eating. It's too easy to mindlessly scarf down your food when all you had to do was go through a drive-thru, place your order, pay and get your bag of food handed to you. Something that takes such little effort doesn't necessarily demand respect, does it? When you can pull your dinner out of the freezer and microwave it for four minutes, it's tough to imagine many folks sitting down to a dinner table without distraction and savoring each bite. It often takes less time to eat the microwaved food than it takes to heat it up. The respect for the process is lost. Ultimately, the respect for ourselves is lost.

That's a big statement, I know. But with lack of respect for food, comes overeating, probably mostly due to mindless eating. With overeating comes weight gain and/or self-loathing. With lower self-esteem, comes the lack of desire to present oneself well. Less attention to detail breeds disorder. Disorder leads to a cluttered environment. Next thing you know you wake up in a messy apartment that you don't have the energy to clean. This is depressing, so you reach for food... the food you lack respect for... and repeat the whole process. 'So what are you saying Jule? Are you saying that respect for self can be born from learning to respect food?' I think I am. At least that is how it unfolded for me. If you are being mindful in life, you can see how your behaviors and habits are linked together.

I noticed that lack of respect in general was a problem that seeped into many areas of my life. We take care of that which we respect. I didn't respect me... I didn't take care of me. I didn't honor my needs and wants. I didn't care about how I presented myself. I didn't do my hair or makeup. Didn't buy flattering clothes. Didn't clean my immediate environment. Didn't give myself my alone time. Didn't exercise enough to keep my body strong. Didn't make sure I got enough sleep. It's a vicious cycle that feeds into itself, creating more chaos and more negative behaviors. This goes back to my Tilt-A-Whirl.

The things we care about most are what we put our efforts into. For some reason I got a vision of a man in his driveway polishing his shiny sports car. He is taking time to make it look great, even though it already looks darn good, because he holds it in high regard. He may spend hours admiring it, cleaning and polishing and starting all over when he is through. Some may feel that is excessive, but if he respects and essentially loves his car he is going to take good care of it and invest the time it takes to give such good care. We need to start caring for ourselves and investing the time in ourselves. Exercise is one of the main things I believe can help you respect yourself, which brings us to the next chapter.

Chapter 15
Get Moving!

Many of us live completely sedentary lives. We go to work, sit at a desk all day, then come home and sit as often as we can when we get there. Yes, we are tired. Yes, we work hard and deserve to sit and relax, but many of us watch an extraordinary amount of television, or spend our time hooked up to our computers and cell phones. Likewise, children spend all day in school sitting, and often watching TV, playing on the computer, spending time on their phones, or playing video games. We all spend way too much time not moving!

It would be great if we could spend hours each day dedicated to exercising, but for most of us that is unrealistic. Many people don't enjoy exercise, don't think they can do it, or understand where to begin. The idea of starting a formal exercise program may be too overwhelming. But, if you get off the couch or off your favorite chair more often, you will burn more calories and find yourself feeling stronger. Simply start by moving more.

Opportunities to move more present themselves all day. For example, I worked in a large medical center. I parked about one quarter mile away from my office. I could have chosen to take the shuttle, but instead I walked to the office. I got a half-mile walk every day getting to and from my car. I take the stairs whenever possible. If you never take the stairs, start with one flight at a time. If you get a half hour lunch break, walk for ten or fifteen minutes first, and then eat your lunch. Set up walking dates after work with coworkers, friends or neighbors. If you don't have anyone who would like to go with you, you could look in your community and see if there are any groups you can join that revolve around physical activity.

You will move more often if one of your focuses is keeping a clean home. This goes back to respecting yourself and investing the time to do so. Clutter often creates anxiety. Many of us, especially when we have tendencies towards depression/anxiety, tend not to keep our places neat. This can create a vicious cycle. The more clutter, the more depressed you become, the less you want to clean up your clutter. When you get home from work, if you spend an hour or so straightening up, you will get more movement in and end up with an environment that is more pleasant. The more pleasant your immediate environment, the calmer you will feel, the more likely you will keep your tendencies towards emotional eating in check. Having a neat, clean home takes a lot of work, which burns calories, but it also gives you more motivation to do more. It can help give you a sense of pride, which helps build confidence.

The argument many people give is that they are too tired to cook and clean, and especially too tired to exercise. If you are heavy it does take a lot of energy to move. I believe that you are tired. At 350 pounds, I was exhausted. But, there is no way to get extra energy to do the things you want to do until you start moving more, no matter how hard it is. You have to understand that you are worth the effort and force yourself to do it. It is not easy. I don't want to sugarcoat it… it may not get easier for a while. ***But, before you know it, you'll be doing things you never thought you could do.*** At one point, it was all I could do to get off the couch and do the dishes. My back would ache leaning over the sink and the very thought of doing it was exhausting. The person I was at that time would have never believed that I would run again or climb over huge rocks during a hike.

You may have physical limitations right now, but don't let your emotional or mental limitations hold you back as well. You can do a lot more than you think you can!

Reduce Screen Time

You can start by keeping your screen time down to a couple of hours per day. Your screen time is the time spent in front of the TV, laptop, tablet, or phone. To many people this will sound ridiculous. There is so much on TV these days, hundreds of shows and movies you can watch. Many ways to watch too, like streaming or renting cheap movies from the box. There are some people who watch TV as soon as they wake up and as soon as they get home from work until they go to bed. Some people are glued to their computers and phones. Do yourself a favor and take a few days to step back and log how many screen hours you put in. Whatever number that is, which may be higher than you think, start by decreasing it an hour per day and trying to fill that time with some activity that takes movement. You can also use some screen time wisely. When you are watching TV, you can do resistance exercises and stretch. That's even better!

Start Exercising Intentionally

Many people cringe when you tell them they should exercise. All these excuses start flying out of their mouths. I don't have time. I'm too tired. I don't have a babysitter. I don't know what to do. I can't afford to join a gym. The list goes on and on. The truth is none of us can afford not to exercise. Our bodies were meant to move. They need to move. Your body will thank you.

If you have time to watch three hours of TV a week, then that is three hours a week you could be exercising. Let your family and friends know it is a priority. If you feel like your children would get in the way, tell them it is time for their exercise too. Young children love to imitate their parents. Put on music and march around the house and I bet they will march right behind you. You will be getting fit while teaching them the importance of fitness. It will be good for them to get off the couch too!

It is especially important to exercise if you have insulin resistance or diabetes. If you are overweight, it is likely you have some degree of insulin resistance. The more exercise you do, the more efficiently your body can use your insulin to help your blood sugar get into your cells to be burned for energy. Also, muscle burns more calories at rest than fat. Your body can use more calories throughout the day if you have more muscle mass, even if you are sitting around relaxing. That's good news for those of us who have weight to lose but like to eat!

Benefits of Exercise:

- More stamina for everyday activities.
- Lose body fat.
- Build muscle, which increases metabolism (A pound of muscle burns about 60 calories a day while a pound of fat burns 5.).
- Helps you sleep
- Reduces stress
- Helps relieve symptoms of depression, anxiety, and PMS by increasing endorphins and serotonin, those "feel good" chemicals in our bodies
- Since you feel better in general, it can help you reduce emotional eating or other addictive behaviors
- Reduces risk of heart disease and some cancers
- Improves insulin action
- Makes you feel healthier so you make healthier choices

Proper Footwear

Make sure you have the proper footwear. Our foundation starts at our feet. Having enough room for our toes and feet to spread out will make our gait better. Moving with the proper stride and having your feet planted firmly, with an even distribution of pressure can help prevent injury. I recommend going to your local sneaker store and asking them to fit you for a good athletic shoe. Tell them what your goals are and what your price range is and they will help you select the proper shoe for you. The store in my neighborhood watches you walk or run (if that is your goal) to make sure you are putting even pressure and not rolling in or out, which puts more strain on your joints.

A Few Words On Hygiene

Please wear the proper clothing. It needs to be loose enough for comfort, but tight enough that it gives you support and keeps your skin from rubbing on skin. They have material now that wicks sweat away from your body. It is definitely a good investment. There are "generic" workout clothes with wicking material so you don't have to spend big bucks on name brands. Getting a little more personal... take off your sweaty clothes as soon as possible after you exercise. You need to clean thoroughly in your cracks and crevices and make sure to dry off well.

It is important to do all these things. I know from experience:

8.15.06

This summer it was muggy and hot. I was exercising harder than I had in years. I wore loose clothes, so I thought that would keep my skin healthy. My bikini line got so itchy one night I thought it was on fire. The only thing that made me feel better was icing it. I put diaper rash ointment on the area and it didn't get

better after a week. I called my doctor and she
ordered an anti-fungal cream. Of course I wasn't
smart enough to take time off from the particular
exercise that gave me the chafing. [Allow your
body to heal!] A week after my bikini line healed
I got an infection under my lower abdomen fat
roll. It was a four-inch by two-inch strip of raw
skin. I didn't notice it had happened. It didn't
hurt. Now I make it a habit of looking at my skin
after I shower to make sure I don't have any
problem areas.

I always showered when I was done exercising, but I never
waited until I cooled down enough. If you are hot from exercise and
then you take a warm shower, you will keep sweating, especially in
the skin folds. Now I wait until I'm definitely cooled down before I
shower. I make sure all the moisture is gone. If I have any problem
areas, I put cornstarch powder on afterwards to absorb any excess
moisture. If I can't shower soon after I exercise, I change my clothes
to get into something dry, especially my undergarments. I also use
baby wipes in certain areas to help get rid of bacteria. I know it's a
gross topic, but you must make sure you don't let your skin get
irritated. If you do have irritated skin, it's a perfectly good reason not
to exercise. We don't need any more of those excuses!

There are great products on the market now to help reduce
friction as you exercise to cut down on the chafing. There are sticks,
roll-ons, and gels. You can use them anywhere you have issues: in
skin folds, the insides of your arms or thighs, creases where your
clothing or undergarments rub, etc. The more you prepare yourself
ahead of time, the better off you'll be.

Getting Started

Before you start any exercise program, consult with your
doctor to let him/her know your goals and make sure it is safe to

start exercising. A personal trainer can be a big help, especially when you are getting started. I am not a personal trainer; the advice I give regarding exercise are little tips that I have learned along the way. Please, before you take anyone's advice, listen to your body; only do movement that does not cause excessive discomfort. You should never be in pain!

I am not saying you have to go out and run five miles a day and lift weights five days a week. **I *am* saying you need to start moving.** Exercise should not be painful. It should not be something you dread doing. It should not leave you exhausted. It should not leave you so out of breath that you cannot talk. If you cannot talk, then you need to slow down or take a break. It should not make your heart feel like it is going to pound out of your chest.

I think walking is one of the best things you can do to start becoming more fit. All you need is your shoes and clothes. You can do it from any location. You can do it on your break at work. You can march around the house in between loads of laundry. Sometimes if I don't want to do any specific exercise, I put on my favorite music and dance around the house until I don't feel like it anymore. It might be one song. It might be ten. Start listening to your body's signals. Often if you start moving, your body will crave more. If you are tired, movement often gives you energy. I know it sounds backwards, but try moving next time you want to take a nap. It could be that your body is craving increased heart rate and oxygen circulation, not necessarily that it needs rest.

Use the ten-minute rule: if after ten minutes of exercise your body is telling you to stop, then stop. More often than not, I bet you will find you'd like to keep going.

Warm Up, Cool Down, and Stretching

Our muscles stretch and contract to do their jobs. If we warm our muscles up before we exercise, they will be better prepared to do the work. If you stretch regularly as a part of your exercise routine, your muscles will be more flexible and perform better. Warming up, stretching, and cooling down will help to prevent injury.

If you choose to walk for ten minutes as your activity, you can walk at a slower pace for a couple minutes, walk more briskly for the next six, and then cool down for the last couple. Your heart is a muscle and benefits from a warm up and cool down.

Some days I feel that my body doesn't want to get going. If two minutes of walking slowly isn't enough warm up, I go for five. If that is not enough warm up, I will go for fifteen. Sometimes, for many reasons, your body may not want to go briskly at all. It is better to walk slowly at a "warm up" pace for a half hour rather than not to walk at all. It is always better to move than to not move, no matter how slowly or sporadically you are moving.

Stretch your entire body as often as you can. I start from the top and work down so I don't forget anything. I stretch my neck, shoulders, arms, upper back, lower back, sides, butt, hips, groin, and legs, front and back. I roll my wrists and ankles out in each direction. You should do what is called static stretching, which means no bouncing. If you bounce, you could injure yourself because you might bounce too hard and stretch too far. If you are unsure of how to stretch, I recommend Rochelle Rice's <u>Real Fitness for Real Women</u>. It is a practical guide for plus-size women to get started on a workout program. It is a great book to introduce you to proper form. You can also find stretches for different muscle groups on the Internet.

Stretching itself burns some calories so it can be thought of as an extension of your workout. Maybe all you want to do is stretch some days. That is ok too. Listen to your body.

I tend to push too hard. More isn't necessarily better. Excessive exercise will hurt your muscles, heart, and mind. It will make you fatigued. You will be upset you cannot reach goals you have made. It is important that you weave exercise into your life and make it part of your routine. That doesn't mean that if you decide to exercise on Tuesday, Thursday, and Sunday you cannot be flexible and change the days of the week. It means that you try to be consistent. It means that you make every effort to move as many days during your week as possible.

I think it is good to set up a routine. For example, your family and friends will get used to every Tuesday and Thursday being exercise days during the week. They will know that at some point you will exercise on Saturday or Sunday or both. They might start joining you. If, for whatever reason you feel too tired to exercise…your kids had you up late, you were working late, your dog woke you up…take the same time you would have been exercising and do something else for yourself. Play in your yard, meditate, or listen to music.

Remember: sometimes when you think you are too tired you would benefit from some movement. It might end up making you feel better since you will get more oxygen, blood flow, and good chemicals through your body. Again, that is when the ten-minute rule comes into play. If you get ten minutes into your workout and your body is telling you to stop, _stop_. You will probably be surprised at how many times your body will tell you to keep going!

Cardio and Resistance Training

A good workout program should consist of cardio, or aerobic exercise, and resistance training. They go hand in hand. The more fit your heart and lungs, the more easily you will be able to strength train. Likewise, stronger muscles will make your cardio easier. You will improve your endurance and strength.

Cardiovascular exercise is exercise that gets your heart pumping harder and your lungs breathing more deeply. There are many options; walking, hiking, jogging, biking, dancing, etc. Like I said before, walking is the easiest since everyone already knows how to do it. You have been doing it for years, now work up to between a half hour and an hour. Sometimes if my asthma is acting up, I can't walk fast enough to increase my heart rate. Obviously if I cannot breathe well, I cannot go any faster, so I don't worry about my heart rate. That's ok, because moving is better than not moving. Do what you can. Listen to your body. This is part of being mindful as well.

When people think of resistance training they think of lifting weights and getting all pumped up. Many women are afraid of lifting weights since they don't want to look buff and manly. This is especially true for women who have elevated testosterone and facial hair like women with PCOS. The last thing you want to do is exercises that you think will make you look more masculine than you already fear you do. Most women do not have the genetic makeup to get "huge", even if they use heavy weights. If you want more tone, you can do more repetitions with small weights. You don't have to use weights in the beginning if you feel uncomfortable or if it is too difficult. Your body weight can give you resistance.

Many people think they need to join a gym and use the big equipment to do resistance training. It's not true. There are plenty of resistance exercises you can do in your own homes without any equipment at all. You can do wall pushups or pushups on your knees, calf raises, toe raises for your shins, leg extensions from a seated position for your quads, standing leg lifts for your hamstrings and buttocks, side leg lifts for your thighs, crunches or knee raises for your abs and back, superwoman for your back, the list does go on and on. Workout videos are great for giving instructions on getting the techniques correct. I suggest renting some so you can find out which ones you like. Also, there are websites and YouTube videos that you can use to learn about exercise and proper form. Again, having some sessions with a personal trainer can be of great benefit, especially in the beginning of your fitness journey. They can teach you different ways to become stronger and create workouts specific to your needs.

Proper Form

Proper form while exercising is extremely important. Our bodies are meant to move in certain ways. For example, it is important that you never overextend your arms or legs. If you do overextend, you are straining your joints and are likely to injure yourself. It is best to keep a slight bend in your knees and elbows.

When I walk or jog, I have a short stride. If my stride is longer my knees hurt because I am putting too much pressure on my joints. Stand up, pick up your right leg, extend it in front of you and put your heal down. This is your natural stride length. Don't exceed it. Short, quick strides are better for your joints than longer, slower ones. Proper form is also important when riding a bike, another one of my favorite activities. Your seat should be high enough so that your leg can go almost completely straight, but still has a slight bend in the knee when you are fully extended. If the seat is too low, you will put too much pressure on your knees. You should be able to feel the difference when you adjust it.

There are correct ways of doing resistance-training exercises. I mentioned earlier that you could learn proper techniques from books or videos.

In general:
- Never lock your knees, keep them slightly bent and your legs shoulder width apart.
- When doing arm exercises, such as bicep curls or tricep extensions, they will be more effective if you keep your elbows in toward your body.
- Try to keep good posture. Many of us tend to stand with our backs curved and our bellies sticking out. Tuck your pelvis in, bend your knees slightly, and tighten your stomach muscles. This will get easier over time and become second nature.
- If you are trying to do any type of exercise that requires you to bend your knees (like a squat or lunge) never let your knees go past your toes.
- Proper breathing makes a difference too. Exhale while you are contracting (squeezing) your muscle and inhale when you are relaxing it. For example, if you are doing a bicep curl, inhale on the way down and exhale on the way up.
- The slower you do resistance exercises the harder they are. You should not have to use momentum to complete your movement, like rocking back if you are doing a standing exercise to hoist the weight up. You will find if you slow your movement down you will need to use lighter weights. People think it is the contraction that is the most beneficial part of the movement, but the opposite movement can be equally important. Slow, controlled movement in both directions is best.

Add Variety

If you do the same thing over and over and over, you are bound to get bored. You are also setting yourself up for injury from overuse of the same muscles. I stick with something as long as I like it. When it gets stale, I pick something else. I rotate the new exercise in with the old ones. This goes for both cardio and resistance exercises. **Your body needs to cover a whole range of motions throughout the day, so it is a good idea to do exercises that cover as many ranges of motion as possible.** If you do the same exercises repeatedly, your body will get used to them. They will not be as much of a challenge and you may be ignoring muscle groups.

Prevent Injury

Listening to your body is the best thing you can do to prevent injury. Mindfulness not only works for food, it works for movement as well. Notice any aches or pains and give that part of your body rest for a few days. It doesn't mean you should stop exercising all together. In fact, your sore body may benefit from some movement to warm-up and stretching.

I recently twisted my ankle (in a parking lot on a rock... it wasn't an exercise injury, but it sure did remind me to be more mindful of my surroundings!). I cannot walk, run, or dance now, but I can do seated resistance exercises for my upper body, leg exercises and ab exercises until my ankle heals. If your arms are sore two days after resistance training, you probably overdid it, but you can still walk or ride a bike.

As I stated before, warming up, cooling down, and stretching are helpful to prevent injury. It is also important to give your body proper rest (time off between similar exercises) so it can repair itself.

Ignore Ridicule

I have been called every name in the book by people driving by me while I was walking or jogging in my neighborhood. People can be mean. Ignore them. They don't know you. They don't know how hard you work. They probably don't have as much heart as you do and probably can't do half of what you can do. Remind yourself they are probably jealous. They probably wish they could set goals and work on them. They probably wish they could be motivated to do something… anything! If people have a problem with my large derriere, it is their problem. I can't see it, so it doesn't bother me! Keep moving and hold your head high!

Make Reasonable Goals and Stay Positive

The definition of being fit can be different for everyone. If you feel the definition of fitness is walking or jogging a 5k race, doing 50 crunches or pushups, or bench pressing 80 pounds, but right now you are sedentary and unable to do any of those things, you might feel quite discouraged. How on earth could you do all those things when you can't make it up the stairs without huffing and puffing, right? Over time you can and you will become more fit. You have to take small steps every day towards your goal and never give up. You have to make exercise a part of your routine. You owe it to yourself and your loved ones to take care of yourself. Stay positive. Set reasonable goals along the way. Any improvement in fitness will give you benefits. Enjoy the journey!

I couldn't run for years. I missed it terribly. With aches and pains from my weight, it would have been almost impossible to run at 350 pounds. Finishing a 5k race was my long-term goal, but I had to start slowly. When I first started back to it, I could walk for ten minutes at a very slow pace. I could go for about four blocks. It was hard work, but I did it three times a week for a month. Then I realized that I could go farther. Next thing I knew I could go faster.

In six months I was able to walk three miles at a decent pace. If I could walk that far, I knew someday I would be able to jog that far. I started to add some pushups and crunches and could feel myself getting stronger. By the time a year passed, I could walk for an hour. If I walked for a shorter period of time, I could go up a couple hills. A couple of months after that, I could walk up as many hills as I could find. Then after about a year and a half I started to jog. It was more like shuffling, but shuffling doesn't hurt my knees. Remember: listen to your body. I would walk for 15 minutes, jog for 5, and walk for 15 more. Over time I could jog more and more and I would walk less.

I took five years off from running races. The first 5K I did when I started up again I finished in a little under 39 minutes, jogged the whole time, and had energy afterward. It was the best feeling. I was happy and proud of myself. I finished last out of the runners, but I had definitely won. If you try your hardest, you will win too.

I am not saying everyone should go out and run a 5K. I am not even saying you should walk one. I am saying that you have to find something you enjoy doing and work on doing it well. It could be walking, biking, hiking, dancing, karate, weightlifting, yoga, tai chi, swimming. Pick something and work on it. MOVE. Make reasonable short-term goals, visualize yourself doing them, and stay positive. You will surprise yourself.

Fueling Your Workouts

When I first started running, I ran on an empty stomach. Like many people, I thought I would burn more fat if I didn't have food in my system. I also didn't eat afterwards. I thought that I would sabotage all the hard work I had done to burn those calories. That was exactly opposite of what we should do!

Now I know I need to fuel my body before a workout. I need "gas in the tank" to go. I eat something within an hour of exercise, like peanut butter toast, a handful of nuts and raisins, or a banana and milk. Your body will be happy to have some carbs, protein, and fat in its system. They break down at different rates to give you extended energy. When you properly fuel your workouts, you will be able to do more.

Your body does the best it can to keep your blood sugar in a tight range. Your body stores glucose in a big molecule called glycogen. It strings the glucose units together in little branches so that they can be clipped off when your blood sugar drops. When you exercise, you deplete your glucose storage in your muscles and your liver. That is why it is so important to consume some carbs after your workout. It can rebuild your glycogen so you can have it there for next time you exercise. Having adequate glycogen stored is like having a reserve tank of gas.

When you do resistance training you create little tears in your muscle tissue, which is made of protein. Your body gets stronger by taking the amino acids from protein that you eat or drink to rebuild the muscle tissue you broke down during your workout. If you don't eat protein immediately after the workout, you are not going to build muscle mass.

I usually consume a shake that I make out of whey protein and milk within a half hour of my workout. A minimum of 20 grams of protein should be consumed within 30 minutes of exercise, especially resistance training. I take my shake to the gym and start drinking it as I stretch and cool down. You can use whatever milk you like, including soy or almond. I tend to use chocolate milk, especially if I know I will be working out hard. It has extra sugar so it can help rebuild my glycogen. Plus, it tastes good!

This fueling section reminds me of another one of my uncles:

"You can't run the Titanic on a Tic-Tac, Jooge" – Uncle Tom

Jooge is another one of my nicknames. Uncle Tom is exactly right… the bigger you are, the more fuel you need to move your body. A lot of people are surprised at how much I eat, but I'm a bigger woman, with a lot of muscle mass, and I do a lot of movement. I need that fuel! I let my hunger be my guide. The more I move, the hungrier I get, the more I eat. And this has kept my weight stable for years.

Stay Motivated

Every day you have the choice to move or not to move. It's your decision. Given all the benefits, you know it is worth the effort. I know… it's hard. The things you value most in life are often the things you worked hardest for. Working towards good health is difficult, but it's the most important thing we can do for ourselves. So, how do you stay motivated? Here's how I do it:

- I remind myself every day how good I feel when I exercise regularly and how bad I feel when I don't.
- I have friends that remind me too.
- I have friends that I make plans to workout with to help keep me accountable.
- I remind myself that I do not want to develop diabetes or heart disease.
- I remind myself that my mood is better when I exercise. My PMS isn't as bad. Everyone in my life sure appreciates that!
- I remind myself that I walk taller and feel stronger when I exercise.
- I remind myself how good I feel about myself when I reach my fitness goals.

- I reward myself for reaching my goals, usually with new workout clothes, workout videos or equipment, bubble bath, foot soak, or a massage.
- Periodically throughout the day I think about the time I'm going to exercise and what I will be doing. I visualize myself being strong, using proper form, and relaxing with my stretching and cool down.
- I use positive self-talk to pump myself up.
- I make a specific plan for the week and stick to it as best as I can.

Journal Exercise:

Record how many hours you spend sitting down… either at work or at home. You will probably be amazed at how little you move. How little we *have* to move now is amazing. We have remote controls to change the channels, drive-thru windows to pick up food, food delivered right to our doorsteps, and most of our entertainment is on a screen that we sit and look at (TV, PC, video games, movies, etc.). Just get off your bottom! Start to record any physical activity and changes in your mood. I keep a monthly calendar on my fridge to record my exercise activity and duration. It feels good to look back and see progress over time.

The more you exercise, the more you will be able to exercise. One of my favorite mantras is: **The more you do, the more you can do**. It works for many things in life.

Remind yourself you want to get the most out of your life… you will be able to do more if you move more!

Nothing feels better than strong:

9.29.13

The first 5k I ran was in high school after senior year started in 1995. I believe it took me around 35 minutes. I took a long break from running when I got hit with mono in 2000 and my energy was zapped for several years afterwards. After gaining a lot of weight in that time, I didn't get back to running until 2007. By then a lot of the weight came off by working on my emotional eating tendencies. The first 5k I ran after getting back into running was this same 5k, and I did it in 39:20. Yesterday, five years later, I did it in 29:45 (translates to 3.1 miles at 9:34 minutes per mile). I knocked off almost 10 minutes from my time! I haven't run a race at that speed since 1998.

I feel ten feet tall. I feel strong and connected to my body. *Exercise makes you feel physically strong, and also makes you feel mentally/emotionally strong.* I have been going through such a hard time lately, but continually getting physically stronger gives me this underlying feeling that I can do anything. I can run up a mountain. It makes me feel like there is no challenge I cannot face. I am now able to do multiple sets of standard pushups. I haven't been able to do those in years, but it helps me realize *I'm capable of doing more than I think I can do in many aspects of my life.*

It took me years to get here. I didn't go from the couch to running six miles and doing pushups overnight. The entire journey to achieve the best physical fitness you can will make you feel good. Before you know it, you'll be fitter than you thought you could be and you'll be excited about how your body can perform for you.

When you are not active, there is a point that you reach when it feels like your own muscles don't want to move your body for you. If you've never been there, you probably don't know what I mean. For example, it may literally feel like your muscles are not strong enough to move your body to help you stand up from a seated position. It's like they cannot contract enough to hold your body up. You may feel like you are dragging your body around with you all day. I did. It took so much effort to exist in my life every day. So yes, I know if you are at the point where you feel like you are just dragging yourself around all day, the last thing on your mind is exercise, but you *have* to do it. **If you continue to be inactive your body will continue to struggle.** You have to take care of you. Nobody can do this work for you. You can start by moving a little more today!

She wants me to try yoga?!

Yoga has turned out to be so much more than my preconceived notions. I had pictured all these skinny people who could bend their body in any position you could imagine, packed in a room being all chilled out and relaxed. Obviously, they were at one with the universe at all times. Obviously, I was not one of those people. Turns out yogis (one who practices yoga) are regular people like me. I overhear the people that come to class speak of some of the same struggles that you and I do, but they take the time periodically for themselves to come to their mats and rejuvenate themselves. They come from different backgrounds, age groups and body types.

Yoga at its most basic level is joining the body to the breath. It is being present. It is feeling connected... to yourself, the people around you and to the beauty that surrounds us every day. Physically, yoga is a much better workout than I had originally thought it would be. If you are paying attention to as many details as possible, trying to get your alignment correct and using your breath to deepen your stretch, a pose that may seem basic can stretch and strengthen your entire body. However, the benefits of yoga are far greater than increased flexibility and physical strength.

The time I spend on my mat is priceless. It is time I just get to be with me, even if I am sharing my time with other yogis. I get to feel whatever it is I feel, bring good thoughts and energy to myself, and do my best to let the negative thoughts or feelings pass. It has helped me understand fluctuations in many areas of life. Some days I feel great in my body... I nail a pose I usually do not feel comfortable in and I appreciate all the progress I've made. Some days I'm just tired... I'm not particularly balanced or my body doesn't feel strong. I've learned that those feelings are perfectly acceptable as well. All I can do is the best that I can do with the cards I have been dealt. I have said those words over and over, but yoga is helping me do a better job of living them.

The advantages of practicing yoga are far too many to outline here. However, one of the main things I want to highlight is that living in the spirit of yoga has helped me live my whole life differently. I find myself breathing my way through difficult situations, just like I breathe myself through difficult poses. I can let them pass more quickly. For example, I use time waiting in line to check in with myself instead of getting frustrated that I'm wasting time. I ask myself how I feel and I start rooting down, breathing and checking my posture. I make sure that my pressure is evenly dispersed on both feet, that I have a slight bend in the knees and my pelvis is tipped forward so I avoid the big curve in my lower back that tends to creep in. I stand tall, make sure that my shoulders are back, squeeze my shoulder blades together, open my chest and reach up through the top of my head. I stand so much taller than I ever did before. I focus on my body and my breathing much more than I have in the past, and it feels amazing. Once I check in with my body, I start taking in the beauty that is around me. I focus on the birds chirping or how nice the breeze feels as it rolls over my skin. I am present. I am strong. Everything is ok in this moment. It is a nice way to live.

There are some forms of yoga anyone can do, even if you have physical limitations or other issues. Some people shy away from trying it because they are afraid they won't be able to get up once they get down on the mat. Many yoga studios have chair yoga to avoid that issue all together. I encourage you to reach out to your local yoga studio to find out how you can start your yoga practice. And thank you Studio B in Danville, PA for starting me on my journey!

Namaste (my favorite translation – the light in me honors the light in you)

Again, quit the excuses.

"There is no time." I hear that all the time. It's a lie that you tell yourself that holds you back. There may be no time for exercise in the busy schedule you are currently working with, but if you shift your priorities, ask for help, and put exercise higher on your list, it can get done. I just felt the eyes roll of so many of you, especially parents of young ones, but taking a few hours for yourself can help you stay sane and have more energy to keep up with those little beauties. Think of it like medicine… you need your dose of exercise to be a healthier, stronger you. Make it part of your routine. Your kids will benefit from it as well. They will have fitter parents and they'll learn by example.

I've also heard that it's easier to sit and feel sorry for yourself. I don't think that's true either. Feeling sorry for yourself and feeling bad about yourself is not easy. It doesn't feel good at all. It is easier to start working to increase your fitness, so you can feel better.

What is the key to keep the fight in you? What motivates you? What do you care about more than anything else? Use that as fuel to move. In fact, put the book down and go move right now. Start today!

Chapter 16
Goal Setting

We get buried under our negativity and disbelief in ourselves. We all have many behaviors we'd like to change; we end up feeling like there is no sense trying to do any of it. It seems insurmountable, especially if you have a lot of weight you'd like to lose.

Many people know what they have to do. It's not often that I approach a patient in the hospital who had heart surgery who cannot rattle off the recommendations for a heart healthy diet. They know they should eat less salt and decrease their fat intake. They know they need to lose weight. They know they need to exercise. They know the way they are currently choosing to live their lives is making them sick. They know if they continue to live that way they will not feel better and in fact, will probably end up getting sicker. So, when I approach a new patient I try to help them figure out why they are not making those healthy changes that they know they need to make. Why aren't you doing it?

Is your work schedule too demanding? Are you getting enough sleep? Are you stretching yourself too thin with too many obligations? Do you spend too much time watching TV, surfing the internet, or absorbed in social media? What activities take up the majority of your time? What can you cut back on?

I know there have been a lot of different things mentioned in this book that you may want to start to change. All too often we feel like we have to do everything all at once. We try to change too many things. It becomes overwhelming. We stop the new behaviors. Then we beat ourselves up for it. Sometimes we try again, but sometimes we don't try because we feel like failures and like the new behavior would never stick.

When I first set out to write this book, I wanted to tell you the best order in which you could do things to help make the changes stick. Now I realize that everyone is wired differently, so what worked for me may not necessarily work for you. I do believe that all the suggestions for changes in lifestyle suggested in this book would help you become a better version of yourself, but that doesn't mean they have to happen in a specific order. Nor does it mean you have to do all the things I mention, or that other changes you come up with on your own may not be more important for you. If you keep picking a new goal, make it a habit, pick a new one, and repeat, over time you will continue to become a better version of yourself.

I know this can sound overwhelming because we all have a lot we could be working on to improve ourselves if we choose. The good news is that you are in charge of all of it... the behavior you choose to work on, and the speed you choose to work on it, is all up to you. If one thing doesn't work out, you can either try again or choose something else to try for now. It may mean you are not ready to make that change yet, but only you can know that. Part of mindfulness is not judging yourself. Be kind to yourself as you work towards making these changes.

What do you do well that you can cross off the list? Is there something not mentioned in this book that you have been putting off doing that takes more precedence? What can you start doing today?

Do you want to work on:

- Sleep
- Exercise
- Hydration
- Tuning into your physical hunger
- Learning why you overeat
- Increasing intake of fruits and veggies
- Decreasing screen time
- Cut back on your busy schedule
- Schedule in some "me" time on purpose
- Trying new foods/recipes – appreciate food
- Negative self-talk
- Cleaning/Clutter/Immediate environment
- Clothing/General overall appearance
- Connection with people
- Counseling/Stress management
- Meditation

It's all about changing how you live to start feeling better overall. Your health can be impacted by many factors. You choose which areas you would like to work on first, which will help you make these changes stick. Just start somewhere. Ask yourself: What do I want to do first? How long do I want to try to do it before I look back and see if it's happening? A week? Two weeks? Do I think I can set more than one goal for this week?

There are parts of this book where I may come off as being anti-technology. I do think there are ways it can be helpful. For example, you can put reminders on your phone to get up and move, drink water, or set your bedtime. Whatever goal you are currently working on can appear on your calendar.

Start putting in effort every day towards these goals. Become consistent! Bring your goals to the front of your mind as often as you can throughout the day so you can make them your focus. I like the analogy of a record. It is like our old patterns are this broken record that plays on repeat. The record spins easily and the needle fits in the groove because it is so deep, automatic, and not likely to jump tracks. New behaviors, new "songs" you want to play on the record, have to be made into grooves on the blank record. It is hard the first time the needle goes through because it is carving it out, but once the new groove is put in, once the new behavior starts to stick, it will become more automatic. The new songs you've put on the record will play easier, but you must put the effort into making that new groove.

I have been assessing and reassessing my behaviors for years. There is always something new to work on, or something I used to be mindful of that I slacked on for some reason. On Sunday, I usually think about all I've done for the week and think about what I'd like to change in the following week. Maybe hit my exercise goals, but I didn't get enough sleep. Sleep would definitely be the priority in the upcoming week. Maybe when I think about it, I realize how busy I've been and I need to schedule an evening with myself for some downtime. As you move forward to become healthier, if you regularly think about what you've been doing and how it is working out for you, it will become apparent what you can do next to better yourself.

The Finish Line… Only the Beginning

Ever have one of those moments in life where everything around you seems to go in slow motion? You look around and it's like you are observing everything from outside yourself…. like you are in a scene of a movie where the main character is only hearing her thoughts and the sounds around her are muted. The surrounding environment appears to be more vivid than usual. The grass is greener. The sun is brighter. Loved ones' smiles are bigger. It was like that many times for me during the day of the Philly Half Marathon in 2012. I trained with my new friends from work for several months prior. I was physically stronger than I had been in over ten years. I felt so tall and confident. In the time after my divorce I had to focus on rebuilding my life, and my physical fitness played a big role.

Walking out of the hotel room before sunrise, my friends and I met up with hundreds of other people who were walking towards the same challenge. It was chilly that November morning. Runners were dressed in all different types and layers of clothing. Some with long sleeves, hats and gloves. Some with shorts and t-shirts. There were different swirls of colors in the background as folks jogged by, doing their warm-up. There were people with all different body types. Some runners looked cool and confident. Some looked scared as heck like me. It was surreal. Was I about to run a half marathon? Me?! The girl who a few years back couldn't seem to get off the couch? The girl who didn't have enough energy to shower at one point? Who got tired just doing the dishes? Was I that same girl?

Obviously, I wasn't that same girl. I overcame years of beating myself up. Years of abusing food. Years of emotional abuse and stress. Years of longing for better relationships and not knowing how to get them. Years of being physically exhausted and rundown. Years of not being in tune with myself. That morning, while trying to stay with my friends through the crowd to get to the starting line, I realized I was walking to get to the start of a 13.1-mile race much faster than I could have walked in the past, even for a short distance. Before I got to the starting line I knew I had already won.

It took me two hours and twenty-four minutes. It gave me a lot of time to think and to appreciate all that I had done for myself. I felt great the first 10 miles or so. I was running at about a 10:30 min per mile pace. I felt so strong and on target. Then my ankle started to lock up on me. I knew I only had a 5k left. I had done plenty of 5k runs in the past and I knew I could finish one that day. The pain that started shooting up my leg reminded me of all the pain I had pushed through in my life. It reminded me of how strong I was to accomplish all that I did given all the obstacles in my past. Was I going to finish this race? Damn right I was, just like I achieved everything else I said I was going to do!

When I crossed over the finish line that day in Philly, I don't think I had ever been prouder of myself. I was exhausted, yet exhilarated. As I caught my breath, taking it all in while looking for my friends, I knew that it was only the beginning. It was the beginning of a life I had only dreamed I could have… one filled with strength, love and happiness.

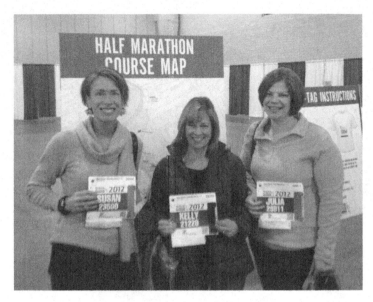

Me and my running buddies-
Philadelphia Half Marathon (2012)

Originally, I thought this is where my book would end, but life threw me another curve ball. My coping skills were tested that following Spring, when life got blurry again. Only this time, it wasn't from my Tilt-A-Whirl... my eyes were the problem.

Chapter 17
Keratoconus:
This Coping Stuff Really Works, Huh?

Keratoconus... another exercise in coping. What the heck is keratoconus (KC)?! As it turns out I have a problem with my corneas. It makes my vision blurry. I also have double, triple, and quadruple vision of many objects, depending on the lighting. Any lights get scattered as well. For example, each headlight looks like it has a bright spider web around it. The lights of Christmas were quite disturbing this year. Before I write about how I've been dealing with it, I want to explain a little about it.

The cornea should be a nice curved surface to bend the light correctly to produce a clear image. My corneas are more of a cone shape with some areas that are thinner that make the light bend incorrectly, causing multiple images. For example, if I look at a stoplight I see the main light in the middle with 3 or 4 images around it that are lighter in color and streaky. These are called ghost images. Everywhere I look I see them.... two outlines of cars on the road, several outlines of peoples' faces when I'm talking to them, letters are doubled – v's can look like w's, c's like o's or sideways 8's, etc. And everything is out of focus in general – trees on the mountain look like blobs of green, like moss, from a distance. I miss a lot of detail – bark on trees, detail on flowers, the grey hairs starting to form on my head, the writing on the stove dials, the spots on my kitchen floor that should be cleaned up...

I've worn soft contacts for many years, but soft contacts don't help this condition because they only drape over the abnormalities and can't help bend the light correctly. Hard contact lenses, similar to the lenses that first came out decades ago, sit close to the cornea and help bend the light the right way. The lenses of a pair of eyeglasses are too far away from the cornea to help this problem. So, I will NEVER be able to see well with glasses EVER again. Sigh. This is such a hard concept to get used to. I've been wearing glasses since I was eight years old. When people look at you and you have glasses on, they assume you can see correctly, but that is not even close to the case for me. Even when I wear my glasses it looks like I'm seeing the world through four layers of wrinkly plastic wrap. I've had to explain it to SO many people, and it gets exhausting. I do try to focus on how blessed I am that I have so many people who care to know, but it gets tiring.

Hard contacts are tough to get used to, but some people tolerate them better than others. I have another issue with my eyes that makes them dry and the top layer of cells comes off too easily (anterior basement membrane dystrophy), so it's more difficult for me to tolerate hard lenses. Even wetting them down all day with drops didn't help. I only tolerated the contacts a few hours a day. They stuck to my eyes, irritating them. I tried a piggyback system, where you wear a set of soft lenses under the hard ones to act like a cushion, a barrier to protect my cornea. My doctor gave me over a dozen sets to try over several months' time. They didn't work that well for me either. The lenses kept sticking to my eyes. It was painful to try over and over again with no luck.

It was quite a frustrating process. It took too long for my manager to hold onto my job for me. She had to put me on extended medical leave. I had to deal with the daily stress of having messed up sight every day for six months before she hired someone else, while worrying about my job and feeling bad about draining my fellow staff members and friends. It was overwhelming. I had to lean on people like never before.

7.12.13

This feels so different from the depression and anxiety I felt after leaving my husband. At least there were times when I could forget about it and get lost in whatever I was doing. This eye problem is ALWAYS in sight... literally. Everywhere I look I see my problem. There is no forgetting it. A friend of mine said "it must be hard to look at the bright side when the light always hurts, you see five of everything, and it looks like a monster." Exactly right!

This whole experience has been an exercise in coping. Coping to me means doing what you can do to deal with bad feelings to bring yourself back to being ok again. I had been in a pretty comfortable place for a while after my divorce. I had learned to do a lot of things to bring myself back to being ok. I read, wrote in my journal, sang songs, ran, worked out at the gym. Well, now with this vision issue lots of the things I did to be ok are not possible. I can't type on the computer to journal because of the blurry letters and I can't see the keys. Handwriting my journal is frustrating since I can't exactly make out what I'm writing. I can't tolerate reading anything for any length of time. Running is tough since I have trouble with my depth perception. Working out in the gym is challenging since I can't see the numbers on the machines. I can't even drive myself there.

So now what do I do to try to be ok? At least I can still talk on the phone. I can keep my eyes closed then. I've vented a lot to family and friends. Most of them tell me they don't know what to say, but even just having them listen and validate my frustration makes me feel better. They are always encouraging and tell me what a good job I'm doing with all of this. I don't feel like most people really get it, but at least I don't feel quite so alone in the process. I can go vent to my counselor. I took some time off from seeing him after my divorce, but with all the stress I'm under I decided to go back once a week.

It feels strange to complain so much and show my exposed nerve so often. I feel like it makes me look weak. I haven't been this honest with others about my feelings before. As weak as I feel, it has also made me feel closer to people than ever before. There is nothing like being real. I've been trying to practice gratitude as well; despite all the crappy stuff that happened this year, I'm still stronger than I've ever been in many different ways and I am so grateful for that.

Everybody has struggles. We can all help ourselves by sharing with our loved ones and asking for what we think will help us feel better. We can also help our loved ones by asking what they need in return and do our best to give it to them. And what we need may not be a big thing. Maybe I just want to sip a cup of tea in the presence of someone who loves me. Maybe I would like to go for a walk, but I'd like someone to come walk with me. If I need motivation to run, I can ask a friend to go with me. I'm also learning that I'm allowed to pause. I'm allowed to slow down. I don't have to run to or from something all the time.

It has helped to invite people into my space. When you're down, you often don't have any desire to clean up your place, or even yourself sometimes. I've been asking my friends/family to come to my place to hang out, which forces me to straighten up for my company. It also helps me make sure I've groomed myself and gotten dressed. When you are in a low mood, it's too easy to forgo a shower and put on real clothes, as opposed to loungewear, when nobody is coming around to see you. If you don't have anyone to come over, you can always make sure you are getting out into the world to do stuff. It's too easy these days to do everything on the computer and isolate yourself from people. Depending on where you live, you can even order groceries online. You literally don't have to leave your place if you don't want to. I don't think it is good to stay shut in if you can avoid it.

Controlling your immediate environment can help your mood considerably. Keeping your place organized and clean can do wonders for your mood. There are so many other variables we can control in our immediate vicinity as well. For example, lighting candles and playing music for yourself can also help keep your spirits up. It is amazing what a change in atmosphere can do for someone who is down.

More than anything else though, I've learned that what helps me is leaning on my loved ones and accepting their support.

8.29.13

I keep feeling like I've never been this needy before. I've had blurry and quadruple vision for six months. I've moved in that timeframe. I also recently had to get put on extended medical leave. There have been a lot of life changes and I've needed a lot of help. But like I said, I feel like I've never been this needy, but it's not true at all.

When I was in Virginia in graduate school, I had trouble recovering from mono, had memory issues, sleep trouble, and developed tumors on my ovaries, while trying to support a depressed partner and teach organic chemistry lab. I was 22, frightened, had to drop out of school, lost my income, had to have surgery, and ate my way up to 350 pounds. I let myself fall down the rabbit hole. Then I let myself keep falling and stayed in the dark for a very long time. I thought that the amount of help I would have needed to prevent it was too much to ask for. Too much to ask who for? The people who loved me and didn't want me to fall into the hole?!

I fought my way out of the hole. Looking back, I see that I fought mostly on my own. I didn't let people know exactly how I was feeling or how much I was struggling. I asked for as little help as I could. I'm not sure why that was. Was I embarrassed that I was falling apart? Did it make me feel weak? I think part of it was I didn't even realize how much help I could get from others, or all the different ways I could get support.

It took years for me to crawl back up the hole. I fought as hard as I could. I taught myself how to change a bunch of different behaviors so I could feel better in general. I had gotten back to exercising. I started journaling. I tried to get enough sleep. I went for counseling, with and without my ex-husband. I started taking supplements and learning about proper nutrition. I researched PCOS and learned how to be as healthy as I could with this hormonal disorder. I changed many things and learned a lot in the process. The one thing I didn't do during that time was lean on the people who loved me nearly as much as I could have. This crappy vision certainly taught me how to do it. Now I lean on my loved ones, but I still feel strange doing it at times.

Lately I feel like I'm falling down the hole again. Every day is a struggle. I have many limitations because of my changes in vision. I get easily fatigued because it's difficult to focus. I have headaches every day. I get dizzy. My driving time is limited to when I can tolerate the piggyback contacts. I can't drive at night at all. Sometimes I can barely read, depending on the lighting and the print. Writing in my journal is very challenging. I have to be careful running and biking because my depth perception is off. I'm home every day by myself living in my blurry mess of a world, while everyone else is at work.

Yep, just me and my thoughts and my blurry world. I spend many hours just trying to keep myself busy and keep myself from falling too deep. And now I'm at a point when I can see for several hours throughout the day with the piggyback contacts, but the contrast is so vast between when I can wear my contacts and cannot, that I'm finding that overwhelming too. I have gotten so dizzy when I take my contacts out that afterwards I just want to close my eyes and sleep. I find it so hard to be productive. To hear the clock tick away… I know I've only got so much time to see that day, and to know that time could run out sooner than I think if my eyes aren't doing well, causes me a lot of stress. The whole process to find the best contacts to get the most wearing time with the least irritation to my eyes has been exhausting. This has been a physically and emotionally draining time.

It feels like I'm falling… but this time around I'm kicking and screaming and putting my hand up for whoever will grab it for me. Know what I'm finding? I've got a whole team taking turns. I've got a whole bunch of people who love me who are circling my rabbit hole, not letting me fall in completely. I'm still doing everything I can to keep myself out of the hole, and I do fight as hard as I can every day. But knowing they are all there with their hands out makes it so much easier to cope with this ordeal.

And help comes in so many forms. I've heard from lots of people who care about me that they feel helpless because they can't do anything for me. But they all do so much for me. They listen, cheer, coach, keep me company, cook or share a meal with me, drive me places, take me out, distract me, hug me, meet me with compassion and give me love. They help keep me strong. They help me keep fighting. I've always known that I was tough, but I'm a lot tougher with my team behind me.

We all have struggles. Some times are worse than others. If we all realized we could reach out like this, it would help so many of us not fall into the rabbit hole. If my readers are in the rabbit hole, I hope they don't think they need to get out of it alone. The journey is so much easier with a team. Even when it feels like you are in the dark and there is nobody around, stick out your hand anyway, sooner or later someone will grab it for you.

The path that my life took became increasingly more difficult. After five more months of this junk I fell further and further into darkness...

1.21.14

I finally admitted I needed to start an antidepressant. I was resistant. I always tell people if they need help, they need help. It's no different for me. I don't know why it took me so long. It is a scary thought... that taking a pill can alter your mood. But, other meds can alter your mood too. The progesterone cream I use alters my mood, so I don't know why this was such a hard decision to make. My sex hormones are imbalanced, so I use the progesterone cream. My brain hormones are imbalanced, so I need to take a pill. End of story.

I really think it boils down to me feeling weak. I have fought this entire year to keep my mood up. I've had to struggle through hours and hours of fatiguing blurry, quadruple vision time. I've had to deal with the pain of constant dry eyes, even though I go through a bottle of drops every three days and use the ointment in my eyes at night. I've had to come up with things to do to keep myself half-amused, even though I can't see well and have a headache all day. I did as much as I knew how to do to cope with this, and then some. I've talked, written in my journal, hung out with friends and family, listened to music and books on tape, prayed, sung songs, drawn, painted, organized, worked on my book, cooked, traveled, ran, cross-trained, done races, rode my bike…. then, all of a sudden, I stopped wanting to do any of it.

It has been increasingly harder to get out of bed, or get off the couch. I haven't been able to sleep. I've spent many, many long, dark nights staring at the ceiling with my mind racing. The tears have been getting harder to hold back. I don't feel up to painting a smile on my face. My skin crawls. My heart races. My thoughts race. My usual optimistic self has all but disappeared. I have no motivation. Celexa time for sure. It worked for me in the past, so my new family doctor was happy to try it for me again. Just started it yesterday.

I've been wanting to surround myself with friends and family. I've been needing it too desperately though. I literally don't even feel like I can stand to be by myself. When I'm by myself I often feel like I'm walking the edge of a black hole… like I'm hanging by my fingernails at the edge of a very large, rocky cliff.

After having to explain my life to the PCP in a short, introductory visit, it seemed even more overwhelming than my baseline overwhelmed feeling. When I got back from my visit, I literally could not stand to be in my apartment anymore. My heart racing, I picked up the bags I had just brought into the house from hanging out with my boyfriend for the weekend, and I went right out the door and got into my car. I didn't even necessarily know where I was going. I just left. All my Danville people were at work… couldn't stand the thought of waiting for them. My boyfriend was at work. I knew I could go back there if I wanted to, but I didn't want to bother him yet again. Nikol would be home soon. Yes, that's where I should go. Even if she weren't there I knew I could find someone else up in Scranton to save me.

I ended up calling Nikol and she got back to me when I was halfway there. I told her what had happened. I told her I was on my way. I told her when I looked in the mirror I didn't see me, and I hadn't for a while. I was to the point where I didn't know if I would ever see me again. Would I be able to see clearly again for longer periods of time, let alone see me?

I got to her place. I was shaking. I stood in her kitchen and bawled. I looked at her with the most scared eyes I'm sure I've ever shown her in the 25 plus years we've known each other, or anyone for that matter. She grabbed my face on both sides, assuring me she could still see me… assuring me I would see me again. She explained she knew I felt like I was floating in the middle of a dark, murky ocean with my nose barely above water, knowing I couldn't keep it up much longer. She assured me I was only in a bathtub with my eyes closed and she and everyone else who loved me were standing around me with their hands out, just waiting for me to grab them. All I had to do was stand up.

I passed out on her couch for a while after she forced me to eat something and drink water. For days I hadn't slept or had an appetite for anything. I didn't shower for a couple days. All I wanted to do was cuddle with my boyfriend. I just wanted him to hold me. I was embarrassed that I felt gross and defeated, but I needed him. I headed back to his place, took a shower, and got my cuddle.

1.24.14

The next few days on the new medication were horrible. I knew I might experience side effects. It made me extremely nauseous and tired. I knew I had gotten my ass kicked for a long time so I was bound to be tired, but this felt like fake, chemically-induced sleep that I couldn't fight even if I wanted to. I had to listen to my body and stop taking the Celexa.

I spent the next few days on the couch "watching" blurry, quadruple vision Breaking Bad and thank God for that. I needed a way to be half-amused for a couple more days until I could try these next contacts. In that time I had told God I heard he only gave people what he knew they could handle, but I was about done. I couldn't imagine continuing my life like this. I couldn't think about only being able to see clearly for four to six hours per day. I couldn't think about doing all that I have in my heart to help people learn to fight emotional eating. It was killing my spirit. My soul was spent. I felt l had nothing left.

I stood in my boyfriend's office Thursday morning before my appointment and cried… yet again. I clung onto him… yet again… feeling like there was so much riding on this pair of new contacts. If they didn't work, I'd be forced to give up my apartment and move back home for the second time in four years. I'd have to think about how to proceed in life with my visual handicap that I would have to deal with for more than half of my days. How was I supposed to help people reclaim their lives and only be able to be productive for a few hours per day? How was I supposed to start my own business, start seeing clients on my own, and finish writing my book when I only had clear vision for one quarter of my day? Deep down I felt like I could if I had to, but at that moment I didn't feel like I had it in me to fight anymore. Could I really get down on my knees again, being more vulnerable than I've ever been, and stick my cheek out again only to have it slapped harder than ever? That's how it felt every time I went to the eye doctor this past year... like I was on my knees begging that the contacts would work, and instead of getting the peace I so desperately needed, I would get slapped instead. These lenses just had to work.

1.27.14

And... they did! These lenses have felt better than any pair I've had since this whole ordeal started. I can see just as clearly with the scleral lenses as I could with the gas perms, but they feel much more comfortable than any other set has thus far. Everything looks so beautiful!!!!

1.31.14

And yesterday marked the end of one full week of clear vision for 12-14 hours per day!!! This is the first full week I can see in a year. It feels like a miracle! These lenses feel like magic. I don't even feel that they are in most of

the time. Not only can I see well, but I can
finally breathe again. I didn't realize how
horrible I had felt until I felt good again. I'm
ecstatic. I truly don't know if I've ever been
this happy or relieved.

Talking with my bud HC just now… we both
acknowledged that I was a woman on the edge of an
actual nervous breakdown. I really was about to
snap… about to break. The branch was just holding
on by one little sliver. It was a scary thought.

2.4.14

The contrast of going from the worst shape
I've ever been in, to the best I've ever, ever
felt in my life has been hard to process. I had
just been so low… so hopeless. I had all but given
up. I had crappy vision. No job. No money. I was
about to give up my apartment. I almost had to
move away from my Danville family. I was about to
lose my mind. Then, in an instant, I got
everything back. I can see all day… from within
minutes of awakening, to minutes before bed.

These miracle contacts happened at the last
possible moment… the day before my friend's
retirement. I had been hoping to move into her
position right along, but the likelihood of that
possibility seemed so slim just earlier that week.
When I went to her retirement party our manager
called me aside to discuss my situation. I had
told her the contacts I had gotten the day before
were working better than any I had tried thus far,
and she said she could wait a little while to see
how I did with them. They still wanted me back,

and for the first time in months and months I thought that it might actually be able to happen. I told her I would let her know by the end of the following week. I also told my landlady I would let her know by the end of the week. I had put my movers, my brother and his buds, on hold until later that week. I was waiting yet again, but this time it felt less like I was holding my breath.

Every day that passed last week my eyes felt better and better. My eyelids stopped being so sore. My eye pain had all but disappeared. My eyes actually felt less dry than they had for the past year. I had been using rewetting drops one to two times per hour and the ointment one to three times per day for months on end. With these new lenses, I really don't need that many drops at all. When I wake up my eyes are not nearly as dry or inflamed as they had been. They are so much less red than they were. It is truly amazing!

So, within one week's time, I went from being very depressed, feeling like my world had crashed all around me, to getting everything back... my sight, my freedom, my job, my money, my apartment, my identity, my sanity. As my Dad would say... Unreal!

It does feel surreal. This whole journey has felt surreal. I had such a hard time dealing with my ghost images, refusing to believe that this was my world now... quadruple letters, numbers, faces, scattered lights, etc. Not being free to drive when I wanted. Not having energy. Constant headaches. The need for multiple naps throughout the day. Now, when I look around, I can't believe

257

I'm not seeing that way anymore. I can't believe I
see so clearly. I can't believe that my eyes feel
so healthy, or that the contacts feel so good in
my eyes, that I have moments when I forget I'm
even wearing contacts. I can't believe the energy
I have or how light I feel. It is a complete 180.
I feel so very fortunate.

Ironically, I see everything more clearly than I had before I
went through this experience. My safety net, my family, friends, and
all the other positive coping mechanisms I used, are the only reason
I made it through. I did it without gaining any weight. To me, that is
a miracle. I must admit I ate my share of peanut butter cups and
Ramen noodles that year, but I ate them mostly when I was
physically hungry. I didn't beat myself up about it either. It was part
of what I needed at the time. Mindful living has helped me survive.

Mindful living isn't about being perfect. It's about being fully
present, being aware of what you are doing as you are doing it. It's
about being non-judgmental. It's about letting life happen, letting
yourself feel your feelings, letting them wash over you in your own
time, and doing your best to let go of that which does not serve you.

I know when another wave hits me I will not turn to food. I
will cope with whatever it is in healthy ways. I think of the habits and
strategies that help make me feel ok as dominos that get knocked
over by life sometimes. As soon as I recognize they have fallen, I
start putting them back one by one until I'm back on my feet. Next
time I won't hesitate to ask for help. Every time something happens
in my life that derails me, I get better at picking those dominos back
up.

I will live life vastly differently from now on. I will take the
time to marvel in the beauty of life... everything I missed before
because I was too busy listening to the negative record in my mind,

or too busy trying to help others stop listening to their negative record. I will appreciate the simple things. I will stop as often as I can to enjoy my friends and family. I will tune in and hear the birds sing their songs for me as I run, instead of only hearing the chatter in my brain. I will allow myself to slow down. I will be mindful, not only of my food, but of my life.

Closing Thoughts

Many people have told me they wish they had the willpower that I possess. It's not about willpower. I hope you understand that now. I don't have some magical power that you don't. I learned how to fight for myself. You can too. I learned how to be vulnerable and ask for what I need. I learned to be compassionate to myself. I learned to forgive. You can too.

You can do more than you think you can. The first step is believing you can do it. You set a goal and then work towards it as often as you can. Taking even the smallest steps gets you closer. Start listening to the nurturing voice within yourself. It will tell you what you need and you'll figure out how to get it.

Look at your life through a different lens. I am sure you did the best you could with the cards you were dealt. Don't just read these words, feel what I'm saying. If overeating or any other unhealthy coping mechanism has been your crutch, it doesn't have to continue to be the case. Don't beat yourself up. Let it go.

When I first set out to write this book, I thought I wrote it for you. Turns out that it played a major role in my own healing. The little girl inside me wanted to know she wasn't alone. Am I? Is what you're looking for in the fridge? I found myself when I stopped looking there. Will you?

Epilogue

After reading this work, many people have asked me what happened to Chet and Nikol.

Chet continues to struggle with depression. He fights it as hard as he can. After several years of searching, he secured full-time employment at a local TV station. He has always supported me, even if that support has had to come from a distance.

Nikol has had a very full life, but it has not been easy. However, she has done great navigating through it all. After a brief career as a Certified Professional Nanny, she returned to school to become a Speech Language Pathologist. She obtained her Bachelor's and Master's degree from Marywood University, in Scranton, PA as a single mother. Currently, she is self-employed with two wonderful children and has been married for over 12 years. I couldn't be prouder of her and her family. Most importantly, Nikol is still one of the main people I go to when what I'm looking for is not in the fridge.

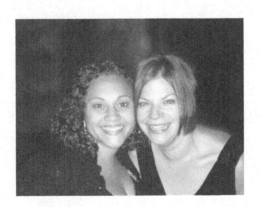

Epilogue

Appendix

Quiz:

Do you have a healthy relationship with food? To answer this question, ask yourself the following questions and answer them as honestly as you can.

1. Do you eat when you're not hungry?

2. Do you eat due to emotions? Sad, angry, happy?

3. Have you ever wanted to stop eating and found you couldn't?

4. Do you obsess your weight or how you look?

5. Have you tried many diets over the years without lasting success?

6. Do you vomit, excessively exercise, use laxatives, or other forms of purging?

7. Do you eat differently in front of other people?

8. Do you finish eating something and realize you don't remember doing it? For example, have an empty chip bag and wonder how it got that way?

9. Do you eat large quantities of food at one time?

10. Is your weight problem due to your "grazing" all day long?

11. Do you have negative thoughts about yourself in your head all day?

12. Do you eat in secret or hide your food wrappers in the garbage?

13. Do you purposely go through long periods of time when you don't eat because you overate?

14. Do you eat out of habit? For example, on the couch or favorite chair at night because it is what you always do?

15. Have you ever hidden food to make sure you have "enough?"

16. Do you eat something because you feel you won't get to eat it again anytime soon?

17. Do you calculate the calories you've burned exercising and compare it to the calories you have consumed?

18. Do you frequently feel guilty or ashamed about your food intake?

19. Are you waiting for your life to begin "when you lose the weight?"

20. Do you feel hopeless or worthless because of your weight?

If you answered yes to any of the above questions, then you would benefit from working on your relationship with food. If some of it sounds familiar, but you don't feel that your overeating is due to emotions or stress, then you may be more of a mindless eater.

Recommended Reading

I have been inspired by and recommend reading anything that the following authors have written:

Susan Albers   Karen R. Koenig

Brene Brown   Michelle May

Megrette Fletcher   Geneen Roth

Jon Kabat-Zinn   Eckhart Tolle

Recommended Websites

The Center for Mindful Eating
www.tcme.org

     The Center for Mindful Eating is a valuable resource that helps educate health professionals and the public on the mindful eating process. When I started practicing eating mindfully, I had not heard of mindful eating. I hadn't heard anyone call it that yet. I am happy that such a resource exists. I encourage everyone who wants to learn more about mindful eating to explore this wonderful not-for-profit organization's website.

The National Eating Disorders Association
This organization has many handouts you can read to help build self-esteem and self-image. Including: Prevention Guidelines & Strategies for Everyone: 50 Ways to Lose the 3Ds: Dieting, Drive for Thinness, and Body Dissatisfaction Handout. They can be found at:
http://www.nationaleatingdisorders.org/index-handouts

References

Albers, S. (2012). 50 Ways to Soothe Yourself Without Food. Oakland, CA: New Harbinger Publications.

Barry, D., Clarke, M., Petry, N.M. (2009). Obesity and Its Relationship to Addictions: Is Overeating a Form of Addictive Behavior? *The American Journal on Addictions, 18(6)*, 439-451.

The Center for Disease Control and Prevention. (2014). *Fast Stats: Obesity and Overweight.* Retrieved from http://www.cdc.gov/nchs/fastats/obesityoverweight.htm

Guerdjikova, A.I., West-Smith, L., McElroy, S.L., Sonnanstine, T., Stanford, K., Keck, PE. (2007). Emotional Eating and Emotional Eating Alternatives in Subjects Undergoing Bariatric Surgery. *Obesity Surgery, 17*, 1091-1096.

McQuillan, S. (2004) Psychology Today: Breaking the Bonds of Food Addiction. NY, NY: Penguin Group.

Nakken, C. (1996) The Addictive Personality: Understanding the Addictive Process and Compulsive Behavior. Center City, MN: Hazelden Publishing.

Ozier, A.D., Kendrick, O.W., Leeper, J.D., Knol, L.L., Perko, M., Burnham, J. (2008) Overweight and Obesity are Associated with Emotion- and Stress-Related Eating as Measured by the Eating and Appraisal Due to Emotions and Stress Questionnaire. *The Journal of the American Dietetic Association, 108*, 49-58.

PCOS Awareness Association can be found at www.pcosaa.org.

PCOS Foundation can be found at www.pcosfoundation.org.

Rice, R. (2009) *Real Fitness for Real Women: A Unique Workout Program for the Plus-size Woman.*

Twerski, A.J. (1997) *Addictive Thinking: Understanding Self-deception*, Hazelden Publishing, Center City, MN.

Vliet, E.L. (2000) *Screaming to be Heard: Hormonal Connections Women Suspect and Doctors Still Ignore*. M. Evans & Company; Completely Revised and Expanded edition.

About the Author

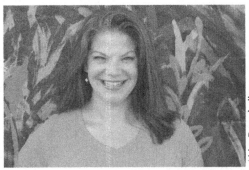

Abby Drumheller

Julia Grocki embraces every opportunity to share her personal and professional experiences with disordered eating in clinical and community settings. While earning her Master's in Chemistry from the University of Virginia, she identified herself as an emotional eater. After repairing her relationship with food and herself, she lost over 130 pounds and alleviated many health issues. Her passion to help others achieve better health inspired her to become a Registered Dietitian Nutritionist and motivational speaker. She completed her dietetic coursework and a Master of Science in Nutrition & Dietetics at Marywood University in Scranton, PA, while teaching in the Science and Nutrition Departments. Julia performed as a Clinical Dietitian at Geisinger Medical Center in Danville, PA for five years. She started her private practice, New Beginning Nutrition Counseling, LLC in Berwick, PA in 2016.